査読者が教える

採用される医学論文の書き方

●著 ………… 森本 剛

中山書店

はじめに ── 本書の目的

　この本を手にされた方の多くは何らかの形で論文を書かれていると思います．その中で，多くの皆さんは，おそらく論文の書き方をフォーマルに学んだことはないのではないかと思います．これまで，論文を書かれたことのある皆さんは「他人の論文を読んだり」「先輩のドラフトを見せてもらったり」して学んだというのがほとんどではないでしょうか．

　筆者は，日常的に臨床研究者，特に「若手」や論文を書くのが「初めての人」の論文をチェックする機会が多くあります．そうして論文をチェックしていると，初めて論文を書く人に共通の，ある一定のパターンがあることに気づきました．それらをまとめることで，これから論文を書こうとする皆さんにとって便利なのではないかと考え，今回1冊の本にしました．

　アメリカ心臓病学会誌JACC（Journal of the American College of Cardiology）のDeMaria編集長は以下のように述べています．

"A poor presentation can sink a good study. I do not think an excellent presentation can rescue one that is fatally flawed."
「発表が稚拙だと，よくできた研究であってもきちんと評価されない．だからといって，素晴らしい発表で根本的にダメな研究を救ったりはできない」
また，
"The preparation of the manuscript begins with the planning of the project."
「論文執筆の準備は研究を計画する段階から始まっている」

　　（DeMaria AN：How do I get a paper accepted? J Am Coll Cardiol 2007；49：1666-7）

　まさにそのとおりです．これは一流雑誌の編集長が，編集者の視点から発言した貴重な言葉であると言えます．論文を書く人は，得てして「書く側の論理」で執筆しがちです．そして残念ながら不採用になることが多いのです．

　本書は，厳しい言葉で言うと「自分流の論文」を書いてきた研究者に「編集者もしくは査読者の視点」を与えるための指南書です．

　本書を読んで，査読者の視点をもち採用される論文の執筆の仕方を身につけてほしいと願っています．

2013年3月　森本　剛

本書の利用法

　この本は「第Ⅰ部　採用される論文の書き方」「第Ⅱ部　論文 Before & After」の2部構成となっています．どこから読み始めても構わないと思いますが，もし，これまで英文論文を書いたことがない人やこれから研究を始めようとする人は，まず初めに第Ⅰ部の「1章　論文執筆の前提」を読んでください．その後，自分で論文を書き始める前に「3章　文章構成」を，書き進めるに合わせて「2章　論文の構成と書き方」の各パートを読むとよいと思います．

　何度か論文を書いた経験がある人は，第Ⅱ部を読んでみてください．自分がこれまで書いてきたパターンのよいところ，悪いところがわかるかもしれません．必要があれば第Ⅰ部に戻ってその理由を確認するとよいと思います．

　もし，senior author として若手研究者の指導をしている人であれば，読みにくい論文を受け取る前に，是非この本を若手に勧めてみてください．

　読みにくい論文の原因の多くは第Ⅰ部の3章にまとめてあります．4章はこれから投稿しようとする人にとって役に立つ内容をまとめました．論文は何とか書いたのだけれど，なかなか採用されない，と困っている人は，2章と4章を再度確認するとよいでしょう．ただし，もともとの研究の質が悪いものは，DeMaria 編集長が言うように，書き方をどうのこうのしたところで，採用されるわけではありません．研究の質を高める努力も必要です．研究の質を高めるヒントも本書の中に散りばめられていますから，参考にしてください．

目 次

はじめに ── 本書の目的 ……………………………………………………………… iii
本書の利用法 …………………………………………………………………………… iv

第 I 部　採用される論文の書き方

1 章　論文執筆の前提 …………………………………………………………… 2

1.1　前提 …………………………………………………………………………… 2
1.1.1　論文執筆は臨床研究成功の最終作業 …………………………………… 2
1.1.2　読者，査読者，編集者は，素早く読みたい …………………………… 3
1.1.3　書き慣れた人，専門家に手伝ってもらう ……………………………… 3
1.1.4　細かいところまで気を配る ……………………………………………… 3
1.1.5　何度も推敲する …………………………………………………………… 4

1.2　論文の構造 …………………………………………………………………… 5
1.2.1　あるべき論文の構造とよくある論文の構造 …………………………… 5
1.2.2　論文を料理にたとえると ………………………………………………… 6

1.3　さあ書き始めよう …………………………………………………………… 7
1.3.1　いつ書き始めるか？ ……………………………………………………… 7
1.3.2　似たテーマの最近の論文を 2 ～ 3 本読む ……………………………… 8
1.3.3　まわりに「論文を書くこと」を宣言する ……………………………… 8

2 章　論文の構成と書き方 ………………………………………………………… 9

2.1　論文の構成要素と執筆順序 ………………………………………………… 9

2.2　Table（表）と Figure（図） ………………………………………………… 13
2.2.1　Table の作り方 …………………………………………………………… 13
2.2.2　Figure の作り方 …………………………………………………………… 19
2.2.3　Table vs. Figure …………………………………………………………… 19
2.2.4　Study Flowchart …………………………………………………………… 21

2.3　Methods（方法） ……………………………………………………………… 22
2.3.1　Methods で記載する内容 ………………………………………………… 23
2.3.2　スポンサー情報と役割 …………………………………………………… 25

2.4　Results（結果） ……………………………………………………………… 26
2.4.1　Methods とパラレルな構成 ……………………………………………… 27
2.4.2　Results に引用は御法度 ………………………………………………… 27

目次

  2.4.3 Table と Figure をできるだけ用いる……27
  2.4.4 対象患者背景……27
  2.4.5 エンドポイントの頻度……28
  2.4.6 解析結果……28
 2.5 **統計指標**……28
  2.5.1 平均値 vs. 中央値……28
  2.5.2 ％には件数・分母も併記……29
  2.5.3 効果［信頼区間］＞ p 値……29
  2.5.4 NS は Not Smart ？……29
  2.5.5 多重性の問題……30
  2.5.6 サブグループ解析と多変量解析は要注意……30
 2.6 **Abstract（抄録）**……32
  2.6.1 キーワードをちりばめる……32
  2.6.2 具体的な数字を出す……33
  2.6.3 Methods の分量 ＞＞ Conclusion の分量……33
 2.7 **Introduction（緒言）**……33
  2.7.1 Discussion と整合性をもたせる……33
  2.7.2 書き出しが大事……34
  2.7.3 簡潔にまとめる……35
 2.8 **Discussion（考察）**……35
  2.8.1 分量は　Methods ＞ Results ＞ Discussion……36
  2.8.2 過去の研究と比較し，影響や解釈をまとめる……36
  2.8.3 Limitation（研究の限界）……36
  2.8.4 Conclusion（結語）……36
 2.9 **Reference（引用）**……37
 2.10 **Acknowledgment（謝辞）**……38
 2.11 **Conflict of Interest（利益相反）**……38
 2.12 **Title（表題）**……39

3章　文章構成……40
 3.1 基本的な文章構成……40
 3.2 センテンスとパラグラフ……42
 3.3 日本人研究者の論文の特徴……42
 3.4 英語の掟……45
 3.5 英語の tips……45
  3.5.1 能動態で表現する……45

	3.5.2 短い句で書く	46
	3.5.3 大事なことは最後に	46

4章　投稿と査読 ……… 47
- **4.1** Authorship（著者の資格） ……… 47
- **4.2** 投稿先（ターゲットジャーナル）の決定 ……… 48
- **4.3** 投稿の仕方 ……… 48
- **4.4** "Not acceptable for publication in its present form…"はチャンス！ ……… 50
- **4.5** "Statistical Reviewer"はビッグチャンス！ ……… 51
- **4.6** Rejection（却下）となったら ……… 51
- **4.7** Rejection だが姉妹誌に推薦されたら ……… 51
- **4.8** 査読者が困る論文 ……… 52
- **4.9** 書き方に関する論文の Rejection（却下）理由 ……… 53
  - 4.9.1 査読者からの却下理由 ……… 53
  - 4.9.2 編集者からの却下理由 ……… 53

第II部　論文 Before & After

1編　不必要な言葉はいらない / 同じ意味の言葉は続けない /
用語は統一する ……… 56

2編　方法は Methods へ / 結果は Results へ /
解釈は Discussion へ ……… 76

3編　受動態より能動態を使う / % は分子分母も併記する ……… 96

4編　表現は明確に /
結論は結果から導き出される主たるメッセージ ……… 132

5編　「何を言いたいのか」が不明な記述をしない /
具体的な数字を入れる ……… 150

まとめ ……… 169
おわりに ……… 172
索引 ……… 174
巻末 執筆論文リスト ……… 176

第 I 部

採用される論文の書き方

1章 論文執筆の前提

1.1 前提

1.1.1 論文執筆は臨床研究成功の最終作業

　論文執筆は臨床研究成功の最終作業である．論文の執筆をもって，研究が成功したといえる．

　「研究を終えたらそれでいい．学会で発表したから論文になどまとめなくてもいい」と思う方もいるかもしれない．しかしそれでは研究が終わったとはいえない．研究者は研究を論文にしなければならないのである．

　せっかく時間と費用を費やした研究である．データがきちんと揃っているのであれば，論文にまとめるべきである．論文にまとめなければ，研究内容が正しいかどうか，誰にも評価されない．論文化というプロセスを通じて，研究者自身が，また他の研究者がその研究の内容や意義を判定できる．学会発表や他のメディアでの公開などの手段はあるが，それらはピアレビューを通じて，公正に判断する点において，論文化に比べて非常に劣る．

　また，論文はその保存性においても極めて優れている．一度論文が出版されれば，その内容は永遠に保存される．PubMedなどにインデックスされれば，常に世界中の研究者の目に触れることになる．

　世俗的な見方をすれば，論文は研究者社会に自分の名を広めるチャンスでもあるし，きちんとした研究を論文として報告すれば，研究者としての評価が上がることにつながる．それをしないのはもったいない．

　逆に厳しい言い方をすれば，論文にまとめないことは，研究者としての責任を果たしていないともいえる．研究者は皆，他の研究者の論文を読んで，それをもとに研究してきたはずである．だからこそ，自分も研究を実施したのならば，それを論文にして，他の研究者に読んでもらう恩返しをしなければならない．少数例の観察研究であっても，きちんと科学的な手段で解析し，報告した論文は，必ず誰かの参考になる．エビデンスとは，一つのエポックメイキングな大規模研究ではなく，多くの研究者が，日々の小さな観察を，「科学的に」積み上げた共同作業の集積である．

1.1.2 読者，査読者，編集者は，素早く読みたい

　論文誌（雑誌）の編集者は，限られた時間でたくさんの投稿された論文を読んで，審査する状況にある．査読者も同様に，忙しい日常業務の合間に，ボランティアで担当した論文の審査をしなければならない．そのため著者の「独りよがりな」書き方とは異なった読み方をする．じっくり無心で論文の展開を読んでいくのではない．要するに素早く読みたいのである．

　査読に慣れた人は，頭の働きをスムーズにすることで時間を節約するために，ある程度先を予測しながら論文を読んでいく．予測と同時に期待感をもちながら読み進むのである．読みやすい文章というのは，読者が意識下で予測している先の内容が，そのまま展開されていく文章のことをいう．

　ということは，編集者や査読者は，自分の先読みとずれたり，方向が違う論文だと感じた途端，興味がなくなり，そこから先を真剣に読んでくれない．場合によっては，その段階で読み進めるのを中断する．

　この編集者や査読者が置かれた状況や心理を理解していないと，論文は査読の対象にさえならなくなる．

1.1.3 書き慣れた人，専門家に手伝ってもらう

　論文を書くというのは，簡単ではない．日本語だって，読みやすく，わかりやすく書くのはたいへんなのに，英語となるとどうしたらよいものかわからないというのが，初心者にとっては当たり前のことだろう．

　簡単な解決法は，論文を書き慣れた人に手伝ってもらうことである．論文は一人で書く必要はない．「頼むのは恥ずかしいからイヤだ」「自分の研究にあれこれ意見を言われるのはイヤだ」などと言っていてはよい論文は書けない．つまり研究は成功しない．

　たくさん書いている人，臨床疫学，統計学に慣れた人は強力な共著者である．「同じ部門にいる人」だけでは共著者とならない（☞「4.1 Authorship（著者の資格）」p.47）．また，扱うテーマの専門家（臨床医）に見てもらうことも有効である．

1.1.4 細かいところまで気を配る

　論文は，著者の性格も表現している．書き方や用語の使われ方が不統一であったり，フォントの種類や大きさ，タブの設定などがバラバラで読みにくい論文にお目にかかることがよくある．そのような乱雑な論文を読めば，仮に研究内容が優れていたとしても，編集者や査読者は，「この人（たち）が実施した研究は"雑に違いない"」と思っても仕方がない．研究がどのくらい丁寧に行われたかは，論文のMethodsで判断するが，Methodsで表現しきれない細かいこと（たとえば，患者に均一に丁寧に説明したかどうか，など）は投稿された論文を信用するしかない．

その際に，論文の書き方が乱雑だと，著者の乱雑さを代表していると考える．とにかく，微細に至るまで緻密に気を配る必要がある．たとえばワープロソフトの代表である Microsoft Word® を使っていれば，表示オプションで「編集記号」をすべてオンにしておき，スペース一つが全角か半角か，スペースの個数は何個か，まで気を配ることができる．

表1は英文論文を執筆する際に特に気を配りたい項目である．特に，英文論文にも関わらず，全角の記号や数字，スペースは見苦しい原因となる．

表1　英文論文を書く際に気をつけるべき編集上の要素

①フォントの種類やサイズが統一されているか（意図的に変えている場合を除く）
②数字や記号が半角に統一されているか
③スペースが半角に統一されているか，またその個数は規則的か
④パラグラフ冒頭のスペース（もしくはタブ）の大きさは均等か
⑤タブの位置が論文を通して同じ位置か
⑥同じサブヘッディング（Patient Characteristics など）は同じフォントや修飾（ボールドやイタリックなど）か
⑦全体を通して同じ行間（ダブルスペースなど）か
⑧Reference ソフトウェアを使った際に，フォントや行間が変わっていないか
⑨表中の位置（左寄せ，中央揃え，右寄せ，など）が統一されているか

1.1.5　何度も推敲する

"Good writing is rewriting" —Truman Capote（小説家 1924-1984）の言葉である．「書く」ことがプロである一流の小説家ですら，何度も書き直しているのである．書くことがプロではない研究者がそれをしなくて，どうして読みやすい論文を書けようか．

よい論文を書くにも，自分で何度も書き直すことが必要である．そしていったん書き終わったら，自分だけでなく，多くの人の目に触れてもらい，助言をもらうべきである．

共著者には，投稿直前の最終原稿ではなく最初の原稿の段階から見てもらう．共著者の資格としてもやるべき仕事である．著者全員で推敲をするのである．

たくさんの人の目を通し，何度も何度も推敲をすると，余計な部分はそぎ落とされ，舌足らずだった文章は言葉が補われていく．内容も文章も研ぎ澄まされるのである．Truman Capote のみならず，一流の小説家は皆，口を揃えて「文章上達の秘訣は，何度も何度も書き直すことだ」と言っている．学生時代，徹夜して明け方までかかってようやく書き上げたレポートを「終わった」と解放感に浸りながらそのまま提出して，後日返却された際，読み返したらあちこちに雑な部分が散

見されたという経験をお持ちの方もいるだろう．一度書き上がったあと，何度も読み返して改訂を重ねることが大切である．

1.2 論文の構造

1.2.1 あるべき論文の構造とよくある論文の構造

　論文の基本構造は，まず引用文献（Reference）の「誰かがやったこと，言ったこと」を背景（Introduction）にして，自分たちで実際に研究を行い，その方法（Methods）と結果（Results）を示す．そして「引用文献」と「方法および結果」の2つをもとに「こう考える」という解釈（Discussion）をするのである（図1）．

　図の3つの楕円の大きさにも意味がある．見てわかるとおり，論文を書いている研究者自身が実際にやった「方法および結果」が論文の最も大きな部分を占める．こここそが論文のメインボディだからである．自分で行ったこと，そしてその結

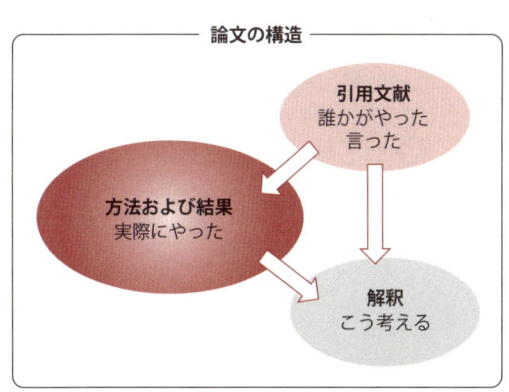

図1　論文の基本構造は「方法および結果」が最も大きな部分を占めていること

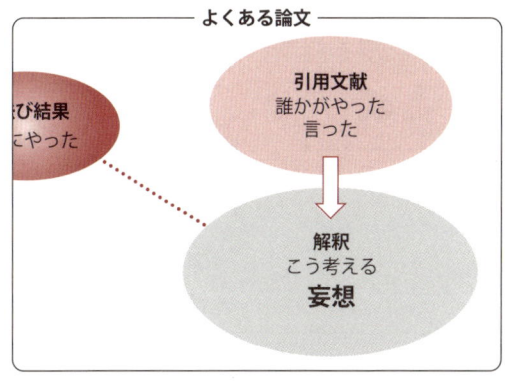

図2　典型的な悪い論文の構造——自分で行ったことの記載が少なく，「方法および結果」と「解釈」にきちんとした関連がない

1章 論文執筆の前提

果がしっかり膨らんでいるのがあるべき論文の構造である．

ところが，初心者によく見られる論文の構造は図2のような形になっている．「方法および結果」より「解釈」のほうがずっと大きい．そして両者の関連が薄くなっている．また引用文献からの誰かがやったこと，言ったことのほうが，研究の「方法および結果」よりもずっと大きい．他人の研究結果のほうが重視されている格好である．

自分で実際に行ったことがわずかしか記載されておらず，さらに方法や結果ときちんとした関連がない「解釈」は，妄想としか言えない．私は「妄想論文」と呼んでいる．初心者は残念ながら，妄想論文を書いてしまうことが少なくない．

引用文献がたくさんあって，方法と結果が部分的に記載され，方法や結果との関連性が少ない解釈が長々と展開するというのは，典型的な悪い論文の例である．

1.2.2 論文を料理にたとえると

おいしい料理には，まずは豊かな農場や牧場，漁場があり，そこから生産されるよい食材が必要である．それによい調理とよい味付け，よい盛り付けがすべて整ってはじめてできあがる（図3）．

同様に，よい臨床研究は，よい研究フィールド（よい農場・牧場・漁場）を作ることから始めなければならない．そのためには，まず研究デザインがきちんとしている必要がある．そのフィールドからきちんとしたデータ（食材）を収集して，

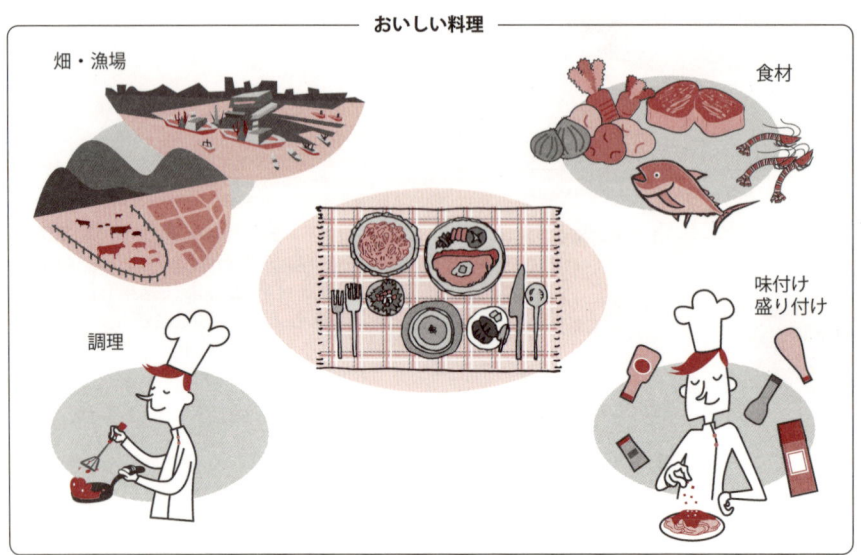

図3 おいしい料理とは

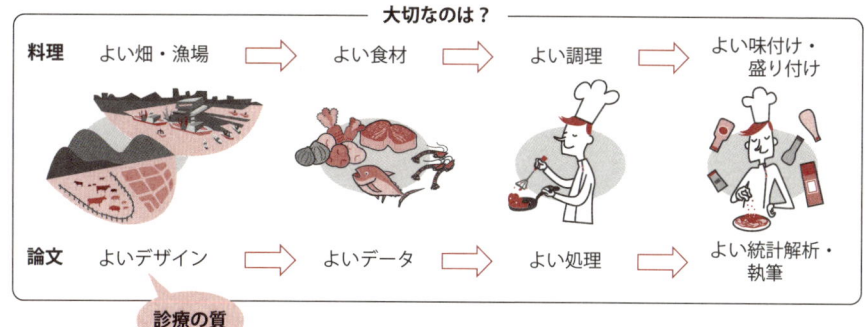

図4 おいしい料理をよい論文に置き換えると

そのデータを処理（調理）する．そして最後に統計解析（味付け）をする．執筆は料理の盛り付けに相当する部分であるが，盛り付けだけを頑張っても，その前までがダメだとおいしい料理はできあがらない．

一流シェフの腕があっても，よい素材があってこそ活かされる．最後の味付けと盛り付けだけ頑張っても，おいしい料理にはならない．論文作成も，統計解析と執筆だけを頑張ったところで，よい論文にはならないのである．

さらに突き詰めれば，よいデータの根本である日常診療の質（図4）を高めないとよい論文はできない．

1.3 さあ書き始めよう

1.3.1 いつ書き始めるか？

論文は研究が始まった段階で書き始めてよい．本書の冒頭「はじめに」で登場したJACCのDeMaria編集長も「研究が始まった段階で書き始めるのがよい」と言っている．「研究が全部終わってから書こう」などと考えていると，書く段になって「あのデータがない」「あれはどうだったか忘れた」ということも起こり得る．論文でまとめるときのことを考えながら研究をすると，そのときは面倒でも後々のことを考慮すれば実は無駄がなく効率的なのである．

① プロトコル作成が最初のチャンス

すべての臨床研究にプロトコルは必須である．観察研究であっても事前に施設内審査組織（倫理委員会，Institutional Review Board：IRB）の審査を受ける必要があるので，この際にプロトコルを書く必要がある．サブ解析などですでに実施された研究のデータを使う場合でも，設定した仮説や解析の方向性などを一度プロトコルの形でまとめるとよい．そのプロトコル作成のときに，論文の一部でも

書き始めるのが論文成功の近道である．

② 学会発表は最大のチャンス

学会発表のときは最大のチャンスである．筆者は，常々若い研究者に対して「学会発表のときはいっしょに論文を書くように」と言っている．学会のときは，準備と発表で燃え尽きてしまう人がいるけれども，もう一踏ん張りしたいところである．結局は最も効率的に論文を書くことができる．学会で利用する図表はそのまま論文作成の第一ステップになる（☞「2.2 Table（表）と Figure（図）」p.13）．

③ 書き始めないと，書き終わらない

物事はなんでもそうであるが，始めないと終わらない．論文を書くことはエネルギーが必要であるが，最も必要なのは最初の動き出し，である．とにかく，少しでもよいから書き始めよう．ただし，一度書き始めたものの，いったん手を休めるとそこまでの内容や流れを忘れてしまって，振り出しに戻ることが多い．書き始めること，そして書き始めたら，常にその論文を意識して，少しでも手を加えること．一通りの完成形にならなくても，共同研究者，共著者に見てもらうことも，論文を書き進める手段である．

1.3.2　似たテーマの最近の論文を 2～3 本読む

書く前に，自分が書こうとしている論文（研究）と似たテーマで最近書かれた論文を 2～3 本，よい論文誌から選んで読んでもらいたい．Methods（方法）と Table（表）と Figure（図）を中心に読むのがよい．たくさん読めるほど研究者は暇ではないし，古い論文，たとえば 20 年前の論文を読む必要もない．あくまで最近のよい論文を数本読んでもらいたい．他人の論文なので，Introduction（緒言）と Discussion（考察）を一生懸命読む必要はない．しかし，その Introduction や Discussion で引用されている文献は，自分でも引用する可能性があるので，重要な引用文献はメモするなどして保存しておく（☞「2.9 Reference（引用）」p.37）．

おそらくターゲットジャーナル（＝最初に投稿する論文誌）も，読んだ論文が掲載されていた論文誌になるであろう．読んだ論文が掲載されていた論文誌とターゲットジャーナルが大きく異なるということは滅多にない（☞「4.2 投稿先（ターゲットジャーナル）の決定」p.48）．また，自然と投稿規定になじむため，投稿規定と大きくずれるような初稿とはならない．

1.3.3　まわりに「論文を書くこと」を宣言する

まわりに論文を書くことを，宣言してほしい．宣言した以上，書き上げなければならない状況になる．また，まわりも「どうだ？　どうだ？？」と言ってくれる．周囲の声はプレッシャーにもなるが，励みにもなる．論文執筆の催促をしてくれるボスや同僚がいる環境も重要である．

2章 論文の構成と書き方

論文は Table と Figure をできるだけたくさん使って仕上げる．仕上がりの面積を比べて，テキストよりも多く（見た目で言うと広く）したい．

図5の論文は，仕上がりでの各項目の分量バランスがとてもよいといえる例である．Introduction, Methods, Results, Discussion, Table, Figure の分量（＝面積）がちょうどよいバランスをとっているのである．

もちろん出版の際に編集部によって Table や Figure の最終的な大きさが決められるので，論文執筆者が掲載段階の分量まで執筆時に計算することはできないが，この論文の比率を目安にしてほしい．

Table や Figure の数，文字数は投稿する論文誌の投稿規定に従うが，基本的に何枚まで，もしくは何字までと上限がある．Table と Figure は上限いっぱいを使うほうがよいが，字数は必ずしも上限いっぱいである必要はない．

一般的に，同じことを相手に伝える場合，より短いほうが誰からも喜ばれる．論文も同様で，内容が十分に記載されていれば，短い論文のほうが長い論文より編集者や査読者に喜ばれる．

2.1 論文の構成要素と執筆順序

臨床研究論文は主に，Title（表題），Abstract（抄録），Introduction（緒言），Methods（方法），Results（結果），Discussion（考察），Table（表），Figure（図）からなる．加えて，Reference（引用文献），Acknowledgment（謝辞），Grant Support（研究費情報），Conflict of Interest（利益相反）からなる．最近の大型論文では，本文中に載せられない膨大な情報を，論文誌のホームページ上などで Supplement もしくは Appendix（補遺）として付け足すことがある（表2）．

表2 論文の構成

Title（表題）	Discussion（考察）	Grant Support（研究費情報）
Abstract（抄録）	Table（表）	Conflict of Interest（利益相反）
Introduction（緒言）	Figure（図）	Supplement（補遺：Appendix と呼ばれることもあり，webのみで掲載されることが多い）
Methods（方法）	Reference（引用文献）	
Results（結果）	Acknowledgment（謝辞）	

2章　論文の構成と書き方

2.1 論文の構成要素と執筆順序

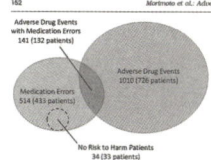

この論文における構成要素の分量（面積）比

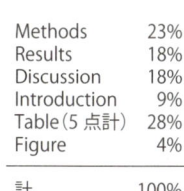

Methods	23%
Results	18%
Discussion	18%
Introduction	9%
Table（5点計）	28%
Figure	4%
計	100%

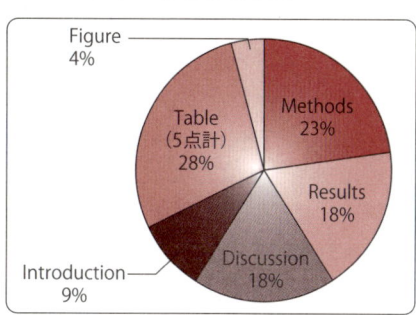

図5 文字と図表のバランスがよい論文例
（論文：Morimoto T, et al：Incidence of adverse drug events and medication errors in Japan：the JADE Study. J Gen Intern Med. 2011；26（2）：148-53）

これをどういう順番で書くのがよいか？　論文は書く順番も重要である．論文の並び通りの順番で Title → Abstract → Introduction → Methods → Results → Discussion と書き，それから Table と Figure の作成をするという人がいる．もしくは，学会で利用した Table と Figure をもとに，やはり前から順番に書く人が多い．

筆者が推奨する順番は，
① Table と Figure（☞ 2.2）
② Methods（☞ 2.3）
③ Results（☞ 2.4）
④ Abstract（☞ 2.6）
⑤ Introduction（☞ 2.7）
⑥ Discussion（☞ 2.8）

である（表3）．

表3　論文執筆の順番
――右側の数字が各項目の執筆順を表す

Title	いつでもよい
Abstract	5
Introduction	6
Methods	3
Results	4
Discussion	7
Table	1
Figure	2

最初に作成するのがよいのは Table と Figure である．学会発表と同様，Table と Figure を先に作ると，執筆の流れがスムーズになる．「最終的に Table と Figure は6枚しか使わなかったのに，最初に10枚も作ってしまったため，余ってしまった．無駄だった」ということも起こり得るが，それは一向に構わない．10枚作ってからセレクションするというのはよくあることである．利用する Table や Figure を決めたら，それらを提示する順番に並べる．ここで決めた Table や Figure およびその順番は，この後の執筆作業の中で見直されることも多く，選び直しや順番の変更は適宜行われる．

Table と Figure をもとにして，次に Methods を書く．各 Table および Figure を提示する順番に並べ，それぞれどういう手法を用いて得られた結果かを考えながら，Methods を書いていく．Table と Figure をもとにすると Methods は書きやすいし，Tables/Figures および Methods が乖離するリスクが低くなる．

Methods を書いたら，Tables/Figures および Methods に併せて Results を書く．そうすることで，「Methods に書かれてある研究の結果が Results にない」「Results を引き出した研究の Methods がどこにも書かれていない」ということが防げる．Results まで書いたら，論文のメインボディはほぼできあがりと思ってよい．

ここで Abstract を書いて，論文全体を概括する．Abstract に冗長なバックグラウンドは不要であるし，Conclusion は Results から引き出せる結論に限られる．下手に Introduction や Discussion を書いて，その内容に引きずられることはかえっ

てマイナスである．ここで書いた内容が，今執筆している論文の主たるメッセージであり，このタイミングで Abstract をまとめることで，ここまでの作業を振り返ることができる上に，フォーカスを明確にした Introduction や Discussion を執筆することが可能となる．

実際，ここまでの作業は，学会発表の準備を行う際と，ほぼ重なる作業である．したがって，学会の準備をする際には，ここまでは同時に準備しておくと，論文化までの道が早くなる．

Introduction と Discussion はほぼ同時に書くのがよい．典型的な悪い例は，先に Introduction を書いて，何週間かして Methods と Results を書いて，そしてその数週間後に Discussion を書く頃には，Introduction で書いたことを覚えていない例である．Introduction と Discussion で異なるメッセージをもっている論文をときどき目にするが，おそらく双方の執筆の時間差によるものであろう．一つの論文で内容の首尾一貫性を保つためにも，Introduction と Discussion はほぼいっしょに書くべきである．

当然，Introduction を先に書いて，それを受けて Discussion を書くのであるが，直前で Abstract を書くことで，自分の論文のメインメッセージを意識して，一貫性のある Introduction と Discussion が執筆できる．

Reference は後でまとめて書こうと思わずに，Methods，Introduction，Discussion を書く際にいちいち引用しておく．Acknowledgment（謝辞），Grant Support（研究費情報），Conflict of Interest（利益相反）は投稿直前に書けばよいが，忘れないように，気づいた段階でメモ程度に原稿の末尾に記載しておいてもよい．

なお，Title はいつ決めてもよい．書き始める前でも，書いている途中でも，書き上がってからでも，思い浮かんだ段階でつける．最初に思いついた Title が，論文を書き進めるうちに，内容に深みが出て，Title が変わっていくことはよくある．表札のような通り一遍の Title ではなく，査読者の目に止まるような，研究内容が一目瞭然である Title がよい Title である（☞ 2.12「Title（表題）」p.39）．

2.2 Table（表）と Figure（図）

2.2.1 Table の作り方

まず，Table 1 である．典型的な臨床研究の Table 1 は採用患者の背景である．患者背景を提示する Table 1 の特徴は，パッと見て，どのような患者を研究対象にしたのかが一目でわかることである（図 6）．なので，Table 1 を作る際にはまず，これから論文を読む人が「どういう集団が対象となっているか」や「年齢」「性別」「疾患の重症度」「基礎疾患の情報」が一目瞭然になるよう心がける．

Table 2 以降は，論文のメッセージに合わせて作成する．ほとんどの論文誌は

Table 1. Baseline Characteristics of Patients Undergoing TLR by SES or BA for SES-Associated Restenosis

Characteristics	SES (n=475)	BA (n=491)	P
Age, y	67.4±10.2	67.7±10.0	0.6
Age ≥80 y	48 (10)	52 (11)	0.8
Male sex	366 (77)	382 (78)	0.8
Body mass index	23.7±3.5	23.9±3.3	0.4
Body mass index ≥25.0	163 (34)	171 (35)	0.9
Hypertension	361 (76)	373 (76)	1.0
Diabetes mellitus	225 (47)	286 (58)	0.0007
Insulin therapy	62 (13)	101 (21)	0.002
Current smoking	89 (19)	86 (18)	0.6
eGFR <30, without hemodialysis	23 (6)	26 (6)	0.7
Hemodialysis	61 (13)	76 (15)	0.2
Acute coronary syndrome	110 (23)	95 (19)	0.1
STEMI	44 (9)	30 (6)	0.06
Non-STEMI	10 (2)	8 (2)	0.6
Unstable angina pectoris	56 (12)	57 (12)	0.9
Prior myocardial infarction	135 (28)	149 (30)	0.5

図6 Table の特徴は対象集団が一目瞭然であること

(Abe M, et al : Sirolimus-eluting stent versus balloon angioplasty for sirolimus-eluting stent restenosis: Insights from the j-Cypher Registry. Circulation. 2010 ; 122 (1) : 42-51)

Table と Figure の総量を投稿規定で制限しているので，常に取捨選択となる．学会発表の場合は，提示するスライドの枚数は，発表時間でほぼ規定される．論文にする際には，多くの場合は学会で用いた数あるスライドから選択することになる．

　ここで気をつけるべきことは，論文の主たるメッセージが，複数になったり，あいまいになったりしないようにすることである．結果が一つしかない研究は問題とならないが，主たるエンドポイントの結果に加えて，他のエンドポイントや複数のサブグループについての分析，多変量モデルなどの解析がすでに完了している場合，多くの研究者はそれらを全部，論文で提示したい欲求にとらわれがちである．論文の主たるメッセージとして，論文全体を通して伝えたい内容（幹）と少々の修飾因子（枝葉）に絞る必要がある．論文全体を通して何を言いたいのかわからないような，複数の結果が並列で列挙されている論文を多く見かけるが，たいていの場合は編集者や査読者に失望を与える結果となる．

　また，学会のスライドで使った Table を使う場合は，一つの表に含める分量に配慮する．学会で使われるスライドは聴衆の視認性を考慮して，行数を8〜10行程度に抑え，それ以上になるとスライドを分けることがある．一方論文で使われ

るTableはその必要はない．最終的にアクセプトされて，論文誌の編集部が編集を行う場合に，一つのTableを複数に分けることはあるが，基本的に同じ内容のTableは縦に長くなっても，一つのTableとして作成する．横（列）は8列までと，多くないほうが読みやすい．逆に横が10列などと多くなるTableは，縦（行）は数行（8行程度）までにしておかないと非常に読みにくくなる．縦（行）も横（列）も多い碁盤のようなTableは誰が見ても必要性がある場合を除いて，避けるべきである．

Tableを作成するに当たって，以下の8点に注意する（表4）．

表4 Tableを書くに当たって注意すべき8点

① Tableはパッと見てわかるということが何より重要である
② 2元変数は一方のみ示す
③ SEではなくSDで表す
④ 小数点以下の％は多くの場合，不要である
⑤ 中央値（四分値）を考慮する
⑥ 常に母集団を明示する
⑦ p値は有効数字1桁で十分である
⑧ 検証可能な数字を示す

① Tableはパッと見てわかるということが何より重要である

本文を読まなくても，何を表現しているのかがすぐにわかる必要がある．たとえば，Table 1で，対象集団を示すのであれば，どのような対象集団かがすぐにわかる必要がある（図6）．この例では対象集団を2群に分けているが，分ける必要がない場合，全群を一列にすることもある（図7）．欠損値や無回答が多く，欠損値がない集団を解析しようとする場合，その解析対象集団が全体からみてどのような患者層であるか明確にするために，欠損値の有無で対象集団を分けてTableを作成することもある（図8）．論文執筆者の視点でTableを作成すると，論文を書いている本人は，どういう集団を扱っているかよくわかっているけれども，編集者や査読者などの他人が読んでみるとよくわからないといったことが往々にして起こる．

② 2元変数は一方のみ示す

たとえば男性と女性で，male ○○人 55%，female □□人 45%と書いている論文を散見するが，2元変数はどちらか一方で十分である（図9）．

③ SEではなくSDで表す

臨床研究なので，基本的にばらつきはSD（standard deviation：標準偏差）で表す．基礎研究で論文を書いた経験のある方は，時々測定された平均値のばらつきを見ようとしてSE（standard error：標準誤差）を使うけれども，臨床研究では対

2章 論文の構成と書き方

Table 1. Baseline Characteristics

Characteristic	
Patients, n	12 812
Age, y	68.4±10.3
≥80 y, n (%)*	1664 (13)
Male, n (%)*	9643 (75)
Body mass index, kg/m^2	23.9±3.4
<25.0 kg/m^2, n (%)*	8332 (65)
Hypertension, n (%)*	9550 (75)
Diabetes mellitus, n (%)*	5312 (41)
Insulin-treated	1203 (9.4)
Current smoking, n (%)*	2604 (20)
ESRD, n (%)	
Without hemodialysis*	628 (4.9)
On hemodialysis*	680 (5.3)
Acute coronary syndrome, n (%)*	3178 (25)
STEMI	1253 (9.8)
Non-STEMI	306 (2.4)
Unstable angina	1619 (13)

図7　対象集団を1列で表したTable

(Kimura T, et al：Very late stent thrombosis and late target lesion revascularization after sirolimus-eluting stent implantation：five-year outcome of the j-Cypher Registry. Circulation. 2012；125（4）：584-91)

象集団のばらつきを見たいのでSDを用いる（図9）．

④ 小数点以下の％は多くの場合，不要である

　％で表示する場合，小数点以下の数値は，読者（査読者や編集者）にとってあまり興味がない．Table中に分母と分子に相当する観察数が記載されていれば，小数点以下の数値が欲しい人は，その気になれば計算できる．したがって，1％（せいぜい10％まで）以下の場合を除くほとんどの場合，小数点以下の数字は不要である．逆に小数点以下の数字が延々と続いていると，読みやすさに影響する（図9）．

⑤ 中央値（四分位値）を考慮する

　連続変数の場合，いつも平均値とSDを使うのではなく，時によっては中央値（メジアン）や四分位値，範囲を使う．図10ではHospitalized days（入院期間）に中央値（メジアン）を使っている．これは平均値が，実際の集団の代表値を外れるためである．また順序変数についてもどういった形で表現するのが適切か，必ず検討する（☞「2.5.1 平均値 vs. 中央値」p.28）．

⑥ 常に母集団を明示する

　％を表示する際は，常に母集団 n を入れておく．そうすれば，読者（査読者や編

2.2 Table（表）と Figure（図）

TABLE 1. *Characteristics of survey respondents according to the availability of time trade-off (TTO) data*

Variables	Total (n = 762)	TTO available (n = 467)	TTO not available (n = 295)	P*
Male, n (%)	386 (51)	241 (51)	145 (48)	0.54
Mean age, yr (SD)	67 (8.7)	67 (8.6)	68 (8.9)	0.09
Mean duration of PD, yr (SD)	9.4 (6.7)	9.3 (7.0)	9.7 (6.3)	0.47
Hoehn and Yahr stage, n (%)				<0.0001
0	67 (9.1)	47 (10.3)	20 (7.0)	
1	109 (14.7)	81 (17.7)	28 (9.9)	
2	64 (8.6)	41 (9.0)	23 (8.1)	
3	204 (27.6)	124 (27.2)	80 (28.2)	
4	202 (27.3)	127 (27.9)	75 (26.4)	
5	94 (12.7)	36 (7.9)	58 (20.4)	
No. comorbidities, median (range)	1 (0–5)	1 (0–4)	1 (0–5)	0.68
No. drugs, median (range)	3 (2–4)	3 (2–4)	3 (2–4)	0.31
Treatment status, n (%)				0.08
Hospitalization	49 (6.5)	23 (5.0)	26 (9.0)	
Ambulatory care	691 (91.6)	434 (93.3)	257 (88.9)	
No medical attention	14 (1.9)	8 (1.7)	6 (2.1)	
Summary score (0–100) of the SF-36, mean (SD)				
General health	34.2 (16.5)	35.5 (16.6)	32.1 (16.1)	0.009
Physical functioning	41.0 (27.5)	44.6 (27.5)	35.3 (26.4)	<0.0001
Role physical	20.3 (33.1)	22.9 (35.0)	15.6 (28.7)	0.004
Role emotional	25.2 (38.8)	28.9 (40.7)	18.5 (34.3)	0.0005
Social functioning	47.2 (28.0)	49.5 (28.8)	43.4 (26.1)	0.004
Mental health	49.3 (20.2)	50.8 (20.1)	46.6 (20.0)	0.007
Bodily pain	49.7 (27.6)	51.8 (27.9)	46.2 (26.8)	0.007
Vitality	36.0 (19.7)	37.8 (19.7)	33.1 (19.4)	0.002

*χ^2 tests were used for gender, Hoehn and Yahr stage, and treatment status; t-tests were used for age, duration of PD, and summary scores of the SF-36. Wilcoxon rank sum tests were used for the number of comorbidities, and the number of drugs.

図 8 欠損値の有無で対象集団を分けた Table

（Morimoto T, et al：Impact of social functioning and vitality on preference for life in patients with Parkinson's disease. Mov Disord. 2003；18（2）：171-5）

Table 2. Patient Characteristics in the Derivation and Validation Sets for Patients Prescribed ACE inhibitors

（2元変数は一方で十分／SE ではなく SD／小数点以下の % は不要）

Characteristic	Derivation Set (N = 1,125)	Validation Set (N = 567)
Mean age, y ± SD	58.9 ± 13.9	57.9 ± 14.1
Male, n (%)	476 (42)	210 (37)
Ethnicity		
Caucasian, n (%)	498 (44)	232 (41)
African American, n (%)	303 (27)	160 (28)
Latino, n (%)	175 (16)	103 (18)
East Asian (Chinese, Korean, Japanese), n (%)	17 (1.5)	4 (0.7)
Smoking Status		
Current smoker, n (%)	125 (11)	72 (13)
Past smoker, n (%)	284 (25)	154 (27)
Never smoked, n (%)	716 (64)	341 (60)
History of other ACE inhibitors, n (%)	271 (24)	108 (19)
History of ACE inhibitor-induced cough, n (%)	24 (2)	8 (1)
History of ACE inhibitor-induced angioedema, n (%)	1 (0.1)	1 (0.2)
Medical Conditions		
Hypertension, n (%)	960 (85)	482 (85)
Diabetes mellitus, n (%)	407 (36)	197 (35)
Coronary artery disease, n (%)	224 (20)	106 (19)

図 9 Table は 2 元変数の一方のみを示し，SE ではなく SD を用いる

（Morimoto T, et al：Development and validation of a clinical prediction rule for angiotensin-converting enzyme inhibitor-induced cough. J Gen Intern Med. 2004；19（6）：684-91）

集者）が自分で % を詳細に計算できる．論文の解析中に，理由があって対象集団が変わることがある．その場合においても，母集団を常時明示しておくことで読者

2章　論文の構成と書き方

[中央値（四分位値）の考慮] **[常に母集団を]** **[p値は1桁で十分]**

Table 1. Patients' backgrounds, and comparison between those prescribed with and without Beers drugs

Characteristics	Total No (%) (n=2155)	BL drugs No (%) (n=1209)	Non-BL drugs No (%) (n=946)	p value
Age group (y)				
65–69	383 (17.8)	226 (18.7)	157 (16.6)	0.0002
70–74	528 (24.5)	311 (25.7)	217 (22.9)	
75–79	537 (24.9)	325 (26.9)	212 (22.4)	
80–84	342 (15.9)	177 (14.6)	165 (17.4)	
85–90	223 (10.3)	108 (8.9)	115 (12.2)	
≥90	142 (6.6)	62 (5.1)	80 (8.5)	
Hospitalized days, median (25, 75%)	11 (5, 22)	13 (6.5, 28)	9 (3, 17)	<0.0001
Sex (Male)	1145 (53.1)	636 (52.6)	509 (53.8)	0.6
Race (Asian; Japanese)	2141 (99.4)	1202 (99.4)	939 (99.3)	0.6
Ward				
Surgical	854 (39.6)	590 (48.8)	264 (27.9)	<0.0001
Medical	1025 (47.6)	479 (39.6)	546 (57.7)	
ICUs	276 (12.8)	140 (11.6)	136 (14.4)	
Doctor in charge (Resident)	600 (27.8)	313 (25.9)	287 (30.3)	0.02
Surgery (Scheduled)	511 (23.7)	413 (34.2)	98 (10.4)	<0.0001
Total number of categories of prescription on admission, median (25, 75%)	4 (3, 6)	4 (2.5, 6)	4 (3, 6)	0.4
Charlson comorbidity index, median (25, 75%)	3 (1, 5)	3 (1, 5)	3 (1, 5)	0.04

BL drugs, drugs listed in the Beers criteria; ADE, adverse drug event; ICU, intensive care unit.

図10　Tableでは中央値を考慮し，常に母集団を明示する

(Sakuma M, et al：Epidemiology of potentially inappropriate medication use in elderly patients in Japanese acute care hospitals. Pharmacoepidemiol Drug Saf. 2011；20(4)：386-92)

[検証可能な記述] **[統計指標]**

Table 1. Incidence of Adverse Drug Events

Ward	n	Patient-days	ADEs	Incidence*	95% CI	Crude rate†	95% CI	Annual ADEs‡
Medicine	1,531	25,734	504	19.6	17.9-21.3	32.9	30.6-35.3	4,148
Surgery	1,469	30,419	407	13.4	12.1-14.7	27.7	25.4-30.0	3,218
ICU	459	3,230	99	30.7	24.6-36.7	21.6	17.8-25.3	634

ADE, adverse drug event; ICU, intensive care unit; CI, confidence interval; *per 1,000 patient-days; †per 100 admissions; ‡Extrapolated from number of ADEs and information from three hospitals

図11　Tableの結果は検証可能な記述の次に統計指標を

(Morimoto T, et al：Incidence of adverse drug events and medication errors in Japan: the JADE study. J Gen Intern Med. 2011；26(2)：148-53)

（査読者や編集者）は安心して読み進めることができる（図10）．

⑦ p値は有効数字1桁で十分である

　p値をたとえば0.0183などとたくさんの桁で記載しても，あまり意味がない．査読者は有効数字2桁以上にはあまり興味がない．基本的にp値で最も重要な意味があるのは0.05より高いのか？低いのか？　低いのであれば，値は0.01なのか，0.001なのか，0.0001未満なのかしか興味がないので，有効数字1桁で十分である．図10のp値は，0.6と書かれている．これがたとえば0.587…と一生懸命計算して書いてあったとしても，残念ながら査読者は正確に計算しているとは思わない．一方で，0.05以上の場合，NS (not significant) と表現されている論文が散見される．これは残念ながら科学的とはみなされない．なぜなら計算しなくても，記載

2.2 Table（表）と Figure（図）

可能だからである．有意でなくても，きちんとした p 値を 1 桁できれいに書くことで，丁寧な論文とみなされる（☞「2.5.4 NS は Not Smart ？」p.29）．

⑧ 検証可能な数字を示す

Table ではできるだけ検証可能な記述を意識する．極端な例を出すと，プロペンシティスコア（propensity score）を用いて解析したと記載してあり，結果でいきなりハザード比がポンと出てきたら，査読しているほうは何が何だかわからない．途中がブラックボックスになってしまっていてはよくない．できる限り検証可能な記述を意識する．n や Patient-days（入院日数）など検証可能な記述が先にあって，それから統計指標が記述されていると査読者は安心して読める（図 11）．

2.2.2 Figure の作り方

Figure も Table と同様に，パッと見てわかるということが何より重要である．研究結果を Table にすることは誰でも思いつくが，Figure で表現するには，Figure にする理由が必要である．

Table を Figure にする決断は，Figure にすることで見やすくなるかどうかである．

図 12 は，ある予測モデルを使うことで，観測値と期待値が合致しているかどうかを示した図である．Table ではなく Figure を使い，x と y でプロットしたのだが，言いたいことは「数値そのもの」ではなく，「数値が合っている」ことである．Figure にすることで，破線と点が近いこと，すなわち観測値と期待値が合致していることが一目瞭然となる．

図 13 のように，補正しても差がないということを Figure にすれば，一目瞭然でほぼ一致することがすぐわかる．逆に，adjusted curve は統計的に調整した発生率曲線（生存曲線）であり，数字そのものは仮想集団の結果であり，意味はない．こういう数字よりも一致することをアピールしたい場合は，Table で数字を並べるよりも Figure のほうが格段によい．

Table と Figure を合わせたような合体したタイプもある（図 14）．生存解析などは，以前は生存曲線だけ呈示していたのが，最近では各時点におけるコホート（集団）数や積算イベント数を示すようになってきた．

たとえば，連続的にリスクが上がっていくことを Figure でも示したいし，具体的な数字を出したいときには，合体したタイプという形をとることもある．

2.2.3 Table vs. Figure

Table と Figure の特徴を比較してみると表 5 のようになる．

Table は基本的に情報量が多く，正確である．したがって対象患者の記述に適している．多変量解析結果も明確にできる．また，数字が合っているかの検証がし

2章 論文の構成と書き方

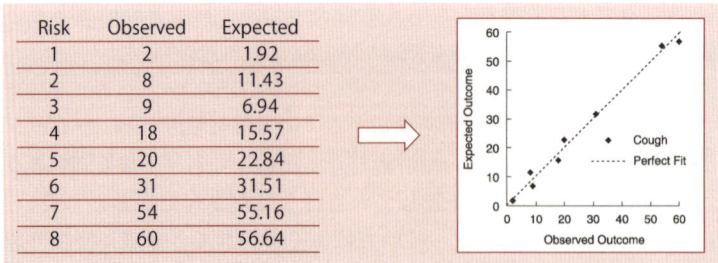

図12 Figure で示したほうがわかりやすい例　その1 — 観測値と期待値が合致しているかどうかを示した場合

(Morimoto T, et al：Development and validation of a clinical prediction rule for angiotensin-converting enzyme inhibitor-induced cough. J Gen Intern Med. 2004；19 (6)：684-91)

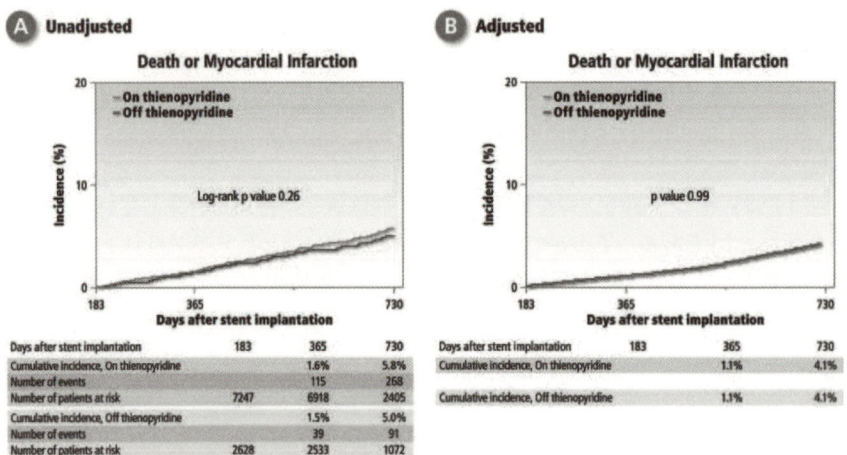

図13 Figure で示したほうがわかりやすい例　その2 — 補正しても差がないことを示す場合

(Kimura T, et al：Antiplatelet therapy and stent thrombosis after sirolimus-eluting stent implantation. Circulation. 2009；119 (7)：987-95)

やすい．

　それに対してFigureでは，変化や比較を強調できる．スタディデザイン(フローチャートなど)はFigureで表したほうがわかりやすい．図14のように大きくリニアに上がっていくとか，図13のように2群間に差がないなどの変化や比較の強調をするときに適している．生存曲線などを示すのにも適している．

　一般的にはTableのほうが情報量が多く，読んでいて安心できる．細かいデータがきちんと書かれているので，TableのほうがFigureより好まれやすい．しか

2.2 Table(表)とFigure(図)

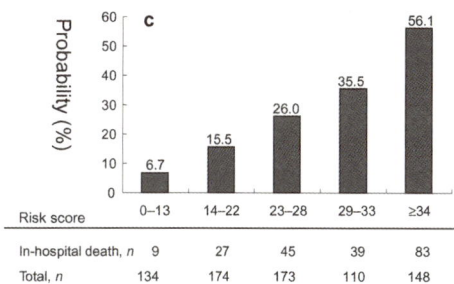

Figure 1 Performance of the prediction rules. a, true bacteremia; b, gram-negative rods; c, in-hospital death.

図14 連続的にリスクが上がっていくことを示しながら，具体的な数字も出したいときはTableとFigureの合体タイプ

(Nakamura T, et al：Clinical prediction rules for bacteremia and in-hospital death based on clinical data at the time of blood withdrawal for culture：An evaluation of their development and use. J Eval Clin Pract. 2006；12(6)：692-703)

し，比較の強調などが必要であればFigureを使う，という使い分けスタンスでよいであろう．

TableやFigureの中の結果は，本文に繰り返す必要はない．読んでいるほうも両方を交互に見比べるのはたいへん疲れる．TableとFigureに書かれているなら，本文中では，そこを少し触れるくらいでよい．

TableやFigureがたくさんあって，本文中に書く内容が5行くらいしか残っていないという場合は，TableとFigureを減らして文章を入れ，全体のバランスをとればよい．さほど大騒ぎすることはない．

表5 TableとFigureの比較

Tableの特徴	Figureの特徴
情報量は多く，正確	変化や比較の強調
対象患者の記述	スタディデザイン(フローチャート)
多変量解析結果	生存曲線

2.2.4 Study Flowchart

臨床研究では採用患者のフローチャートを図で示すことが多い．フローチャートとは，潜在的な対象患者，スクリーニングした患者集団，解析対象となった患者集団などの，対象集団の変化を図で示すことで，最終的な解析対象患者がどのような患者なのか，一般の背景集団とどの点で異なるのか，を具体的に示すことができる(図15)．したがって，フローチャートではどういう集団が解析されたか

2章 論文の構成と書き方

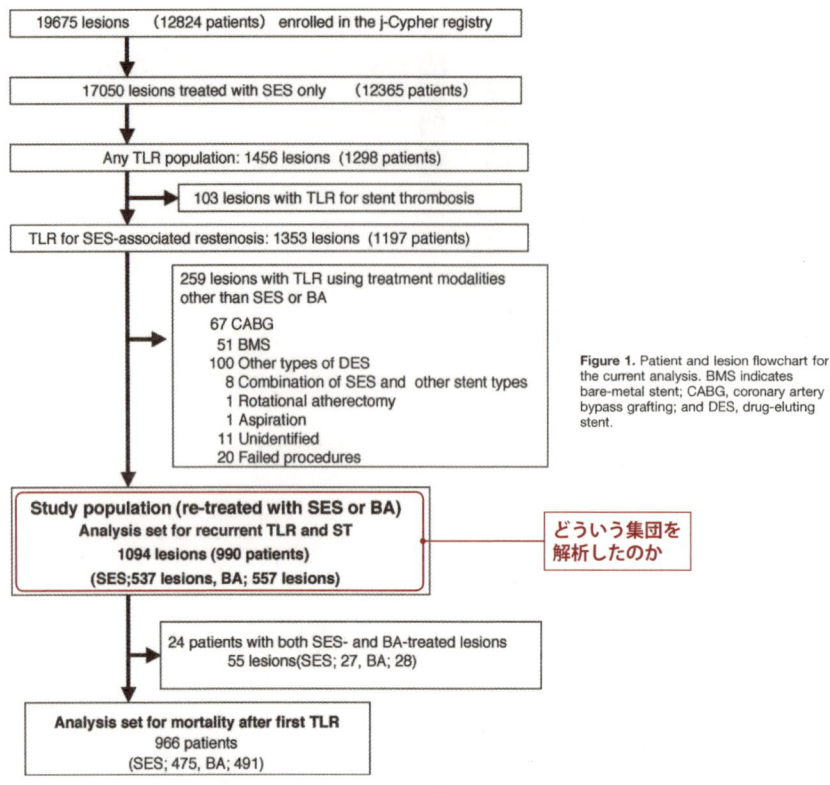

図 15 Study Flowchart には「どういう集団を解析したのか」を示す
(Abe M, et al：Sirolimus-eluting stent versus balloon angioplasty for sirolimus-eluting stent restenosis：Insights from the j-Cypher Registry. Circulation. 2010；122(1)：42-51)

が自明であることが重要である．特に，サブ解析や理由があってセレクトされた患者集団を主たる解析対象とする場合には，どういう集団を解析したのか，どういうロジックでその解析集団を選択したのか，を細かく記載する．Methodsで1～2行「こういう人を選んだ」と書くのではなくて，きちんとどういう理由で，どのような患者が解析から外れたかというのがパッと見てわかる図にする．

たとえば図15の場合，なぜ解析対象患者が最初の採用患者の1/10になったのかのプロセスがわかるような図が必要である．とにかく，解析対象患者選択の透明性が重要である．

2.3 Methods（方法）

TableとFigureが完成し，論文に利用するTableとFigureが決まれば，次は

2.3 Methods（方法）

Methods に取りかかる．

まず，Table と Figure を印刷し，論文に載せる順に並べる．そうすれば，自ずと Methods は決まる．先述したが，Table と Figure をたくさん用意しておき，論文の方向性に合わせて取捨選択すればよい．

2.3.1 Methods で記載する内容

ほとんどの臨床研究論文では Methods に書くことは決まっており，以下の①〜⑤の5項目について記載する．

① 研究デザイン

実施した研究のデザインを明示する．臨床研究論文の多くは，表6の範疇の研究デザインである．まずどのような研究デザインであるかを最初に宣言しておくことで，読者（編集者や査読者）はこの先でどのような要素（例．割り付け方法，データ収集方法）が記載されているのかを予測することができるので，安心して読み進められる．

表6 臨床研究デザイン

比較対照試験
ランダム化比較対照試験（RCT）
非ランダム化比較対照試験
コホート研究
前向きコホート研究
ヒストリカル（後ろ向き）コホート研究
症例対照研究
横断研究
決断分析
費用効果分析
メタ分析（システマティックレビュー）

② 対象患者の選択

研究を実施する施設や対象患者の選択基準（採用基準，除外基準）を示す．選択基準は，あいまいさが極力少なくなるような記載を心がける．

- ×　糖尿病患者
- ○　HbA1c ＞ 6.5％（National Glycohemoglobin Standardization Program）もしくは糖尿病の薬物療法を受けている患者，のいずれか

常にどのような対象集団を採用しようとしているのかがパッと伝わらなければならない．

2章 論文の構成と書き方

- × 合併症のない高血圧患者
- ○ 心臓・脳・末梢血管合併症のない高血圧（収縮期圧 ≧ 140 mmHg もしくは拡張期圧 ≧ 80 mmHg）患者

　この対象患者の選択のところで，最終的に採用された対象患者の人数や年齢，性別構成などが一緒に提示されている論文がある．また，研究時に予定された研究期間ではなく，実際の研究期間が平均値や中央値で提示されることもある．特に，大きな臨床研究データの一部を抽出して解析したサブ解析研究論文で，これらの対象患者の背景データが Methods で提示されることが多い．これらの対象患者の背景データは，研究を実際に実施した「結果」としてのデータであり，本来は Results の最初で報告すべきものである．

③ 研究ロジスティックス

　研究を実際にどのようにして実施し，どのようにしてデータを集めたかを書く．論文誌によっていろいろなパターンがあるが，だいたい同じ分野の論文を見たら同じようなことが書いてある（表7）．

表7　研究ロジスティックス

研究の運用方法
　（RCT であれば）治療法の割り付け方法
　（サンプリング調査であれば）サンプリング方法
データの収集方法
　調査法（対面，郵送，web）
　情報源（患者の直接調査，カルテ，既存データ）
倫理的事項
　IRB (Institutional Review Board, 研究審査委員会)
　インフォームドコンセントの取得方法

④ 測定項目の定義

　すべての測定項目（何を測ったか？）とその測定方法を明示する．研究者によって定義が異なるような測定項目については，特に定義を明確に記載し，必要であれば引用や，その定義を選択した理由をつける．

　RCT に限らず，治療法やリスク因子と生死や疾患の発生などのエンドポイントの関係を評価する研究については，エンドポイントを主たるエンドポイントと従たるエンドポイントに分けて記載する．主たるエンドポイントが当然，最初に仮説設定を行った研究であり，論文の主たるメッセージである．

　患者への質問紙（生活の質など）やアンケート調査を行った場合は，その質問紙がどのように開発され，信頼性があるのかを示す．その際，できるだけ引用をつ

けるべきである．もし，研究者内部で開発された質問紙やアンケートであれば，それがどのようにして開発され，事前に内容の妥当性，信頼性をチェックしたかを記載する．場合によっては，質問項目そのものを Supplement/Appendix（補遺）に示すとよい．

⑤ **解析方法**

解析方法に関しても，単に t 検定や χ^2（カイ 2 乗）検定，多変量解析を行い，統計ソフトウェアを使って，最後に「$p = 0.05$ で有意と考えた」と書くだけではダメである．Table や Figure を提示する順に眺めながら，最初に対象集団のデータを集めたところから，「何をしてこの Table ができた」次に「こういう単変量解析を行ってこの結果ができた」「どういう理由でこのサブグループを作成し，そのサブグループ解析はこの方法を使った」「どういう理由でこの変数を利用し，どういう理由でこの多変量モデルを選択した」と書かなくてはならない．

解析方法で記載すべき項目は表 8 を参照のこと．

ここで記載したものを，必ずしもすべて記載する必要はない．場合によっては自明なこともある．しかし，自明かどうかは，特に論文を書き慣れていない若手研究者には判断が難しく，迷ったらできるだけ詳細に書くことを勧める．

2.3.2　スポンサー情報と役割

研究に金銭的もしくは非金銭的な支援を行ったスポンサーがあれば，その情報と役割について，Methods 等で記載することが，近年求められるようになってきた．最近の一流誌に掲載される臨床研究論文では，スポンサーがない論文はほぼ皆無である．大型の RCT などは，製薬企業の支援がないと実質的に不可能である．わが国では，製薬企業からの支援は「えこひいきをした研究」と受け取られるために，製薬企業からの情報を隠す傾向があった．科学的な方法で実施し，「えこひいきには決してならない」研究であれば，堂々と製薬企業からの支援を提示すべきであり，これは国際的なスタンダードでもある．現在は，利益相反の開示がわが国でも標準化しつつあり，この点からも論文中に明示するのが望ましい．また，製薬企業などのスポンサーが，研究計画や執筆などに関わったのであれば，どういう役割を担ったかというのを書いたほうが，下手に隠して文脈から読み取られるよりは，一般的には好意的に受け取られる．

臨床研究が科学的である以上，再現性が担保できる書き方が大事である．そしてなぜこのような対象集団や解析を選んだかという理由づけが最も重要なのである．その理由が少なくとも編集者や査読者に伝わらなければならない．同じデータを使えば再現可能なのか？ どういう理由づけでこの解析を実施したのか？ これらのことを査読者は常に重視する．

表8 解析方法で記載すべき7項目

① 解析集団の設定
- 一般的には採用基準を満たした対象集団が解析集団であるが，予定していた治療を完結できなかった人をどうするか，検査から漏れた人をどうするか，などを記載する．
- 大型研究のサブグループ解析が論文の主たるテーマであるときには，「対象患者の選択」で記載する．

② 変数の取り扱い
- 連続変数や順序変数をそのままの"数"として解析するのか，順序化，2元変数化や群分けをするのか記載する．
- 欠損値について，欠損のある観察対象（患者）はすべて，外して解析するのか，欠損値が関連する解析だけ外して解析するのか，数学的に代入するのか（その場合は代入方法を記載）を明確にする．

③ 患者背景の表現
- 患者背景については基本的に記述統計となるので，平均値やSD，nや%を使うことを記載する．

④ 単変量解析で用いた比較方法
- TableやFigureを見ながら，それぞれに比較や直線の当てはめ，生存曲線を使っている場合には，それぞれに呼応した方法を明記する．

⑤ サブグループ解析のグループ化因子の説明と比較方法
- 論文そのものが大型研究のサブグループ解析を取り扱ったものであれば，サブグループをどうして選んだのかという理由はIntroductionで記載し，その抽出法は「対象患者の選択」で説明する．
- ここでは解析の中で，さらにサブグループを新たに作った場合は，そのサブグループ化の因子について説明し，サブグループ内で行った比較で使った解析手法を説明する．

⑥ 多変量解析で用いた調整因子とその選択方法
- 多変量解析は上記の単変量解析に調整因子を加えることになる．この調整因子の加え方が恣意的であると，結果を恣意的に変えることになる．どのようにして調整因子の候補を選択したのか，最終的にどのような理由・方法で調整因子を決定したのか記載する．

⑦ 多変量解析で用いたモデルとその選択方法
- 多変量解析に使われるモデルはいろいろあり，それぞれに一長一短がある．論文で用いられた多変量解析のモデルを明示し，それを選択した理由を明示する．

2.4 Results（結果）

Methodsを書いたらResultsを書く．

Resultsとは，論文の著者が自分（たち）で実施した（他人のではない）オリジナルの研究結果である．システマティックレビューやメタ分析，決断分析，費用効果分析などでは，他の研究者が実施したデータが含まれることがある．そのような

2.4 Results（結果）

場合でも，著者が独自に実施した解析結果が主たる内容，メッセージでなければならない．他人の誰のものでもなく，実際のこの研究を実施しなければわからない情報，それがResultsである．

2.4.1 Methodsとパラレルな構成

ResultsはMethodsとパラレルな（並列となる）構成でなければならない．Methodsで書かれてある順番とResultsで書かれてある順番が異なると，読者（編集者や査読者）は混乱する．

Methodsでは最初に記述統計を書いて，続いて生存解析，多変量解析という順番に記載されていたにもかかわらず，Resultsになったらいきなり多変量解析が出てきて，生存解析，記述統計と，順番が変わっている論文をよく目にする．これは非常に読みにくい．査読者としては，ResultsはMethodsで書いてある順番通りに書いてほしい．Resultsの順番を決めているのであれば，Methodsをその順番に書き換える．Methodsを書いたすぐ後にResultsを書くことで，MethodsとResultsの内容や順番のズレを防ぐことができる．

2.4.2 Resultsに引用は御法度

Resultsに原則，引用は行わない．Resultsに「この論文のこれこれ」と引用をしている論文を目にすることがある．しかし著者が実際に研究を行ったResultsなのであるから，基本的に引用はResultsにはないはずである．本来Resultsには，過去に発表した論文からの結果を出してはいけないので，原則として引用は御法度である．引用は方法に関するものであればMethodsへ移し，解釈のための内容であればIntroductionやDiscussionに移動させる．例外はシステマティックレビューやメタ分析，決断分析，費用効果分析などの他の研究者のデータを対象に解析する場合である．

2.4.3 TableとFigureをできるだけ用いる

ResultsにはTableとFigureをできるだけ用いる．対象患者の背景などはTableとして提示すると一目瞭然である．研究の流れやサブグループの対象集団が文章だけではわかりにくい際には，フローチャートで示すとよい．TableとFigureの使い分けは先述の通りである（☞「2.2.3 Table vs. Figure」p.19）．

2.4.4 対象患者背景

対象患者の背景をきちんと示す．対象患者や対照群となる患者がスムーズにイメージできない論文は不採用となりやすい．一方で，詳細な患者背景について，測定した項目すべてにわたって事細かく示すこともかえってマイナスになることがある．この研究の主たるメッセージに関係した背景をわかりやすく提示する．

例　虚血性心疾患に対するカテーテル治療に関する論文ならば，虚血性心疾患の重症度や予後に関連する危険因子についての背景は是非ともほしいが，サブ解析用に測定した呼吸機能やインスリン抵抗性などのデータは不要である．

2.4.5　エンドポイントの頻度

どのような解析の前にも主たるエンドポイントの頻度を明示する．「この論文の主たるエンドポイントはどのくらい発生しているのか」を明確にすることが大切である．エンドポイントの頻度を抜きに，いきなりオッズ比やハザード比，ひどいのになると多変量解析の結果がいきなり出てくる論文があるが，それらのエンドポイントが具体的にどれくらい発生したのかという記述がなければ，査読者は不安で先を読み進められない．

2.4.6　解析結果

解析ではまず，記述統計を丁寧に示す．その後に，単変量解析の結果を提示する．必要性が明確であればサブグループ解析や多変量解析の結果も示す．

一般的には，分量・順番においても記述統計をとにかく丁寧に提示する．何が，どれくらいあったのか，ということを示し，単変量解析では主たるエンドポイントと，必要な因子との関連を見ていく．

基本的な解析結果は本来ここまでである．ここまでの記載が不十分であると，その先にどんな高度な解析結果が提示されていても，信頼されないことになる．

十分な記述統計と単変量解析の結果に引き続いて，研究仮説を検証，確認するためのサブグループ解析や多変量解析の結果を示す．

とにかく，きちんとした記述統計を示すことが，査読者に安心して論文を読んでもらえることにつながる．

2.5　統計指標

臨床研究論文で用いられる統計指標について列挙しだせばキリがないが，ここでは代表的な指標や注意点について取り上げる．

2.5.1　平均値 vs. 中央値

臨床研究では，年齢や血圧などの数字で表現される変数は，ほとんどすべて「平均値と SD（standard deviation：標準偏差）」で表現される．どんな場合でも平均値と SD を使うのではなく，変数によって平均値と SD でよいのかどうかを検討したほうがよい．その他の表現方法としては，「中央値と四分位（もしくは範囲）」が用

いられることもある．
　　例　在院日数
　　　　疾患の重症度スコア
　　　　質問紙でのLikertスケール（1：〜ない，2：少し〜ない，3：どちらでもない，4：少し〜ある，5：〜ある）

　また，平均値±2SDを計算してみると，あり得ない値になる場合がある．たとえば，ある血液検査の測定値が平均値20でSDが15の場合，ラフに平均値±2SDで95%信頼区間をとってみたら，下限が−10などという数値が出てくることがある．その場合，そのまま論文に載せるとおかしなことになってしまう．血液検査の値に負の値は通常あり得ない．

　このように非常にばらつきの大きいものや，分布が極端に一方に偏っている変数に関しては，中央値や四分値，範囲を使うほうがよい．特に−2SDで存在しない値が出てくる場合は要注意である．

　順序変数についても平均値とSDで表されている論文をしばしば見かける．「4段階の重症度指標の平均値は2.3であった」ということに，どういう臨床的意味があるのか，常に考えてほしい．

2.5.2　%には件数・分母も併記

　%には件数，分母も併記する．同じ25%でも25/100と2,500/10,000では意味がまったく異なる．AbstractやResults，Table・Figureにしても，極力%だけでなく，分子と分母も併記するようにする．一方で，他人の研究からの引用であるIntroductionやDiscussionでは%だけで十分である．

　また，%の計算の対象となる症例数（分母）が20以下なら%は無意味である．1件のエンドポイントや指標（分子）が異なるだけで，%は5%以上変わるので，%で出されてもあまり意味がない．このような%は不安定であり，信頼がないので，分数（分子/分母）のままのほうが誤解を生じにくい．

2.5.3　効果［信頼区間］>p値

　p値は「差がない」確率である．臨床医（読者）はそんな確率で医療をしているわけではない．知りたいのは，興味のある変数の効果（影響）がどのくらいか，効果はどのくらい信頼できるか，を知りたいのである．統計専門家はp値をあまり重視していない．それよりも，信頼区間（多くの臨床研究では95%信頼区間）が重要なので，できるだけp値よりも効果と信頼区間を用いたい．

2.5.4　NSはNot Smart？

　時々論文中で，p値の代わりにNS（not significant，有意差なし）で表現する研

2章　論文の構成と書き方

究者がいるが，あまり利口には見られない（Not Smart ?）．p 値を提示するのであれば，その値は 0.6 なのか 0.9 なのか 0.4 なのか，きちんと出さなくてはいけない．このことはすなわち，きちんと統計処理をして，きちんと計算をしたということである．NS で表現するのであれば計算しなくても NS と書けてしまう．また，同じ有意差がないとしても，0.1 と 0.9 ではその意味するところが違う．パワーの問題で，状況によっては有意になる可能性があったのか，その可能性は低いのか，p 値や先述した信頼区間を読み取ることで，査読者や編集者は判断可能となる．

2.5.5　多重性の問題

　一般的に有意差の基準とされる p 値 = 0.05 は 20 分の 1 である．すなわち「真実の」差がなくても，20 回に 1 回は偶然の働きで有意差が出ることがある（サイコロ 2 つで，1 か 6 のぞろ目が出る確率が 2/36 = 0.056 であることを想像してほしい）．したがって，対等な立場の変数を仮説もなく同時にたくさん比較する場合，調整することを考える．

2.5.6　サブグループ解析と多変量解析は要注意

　臨床研究論文で頻用されるサブグループ解析と多変量解析は再現性があるか，常に注意が必要である．よく言われることであるが，サブグループ解析や多変量解析をやりすぎると，単に有意差のある変数やモデルを探したような印象を査読者はもつので，これらの解析を実施して報告する場合には，常に「慎重に」というのが統計の原則である．

　サブグループ解析や多変量解析を行う際の注意点は，以下の通りである．

(1) サブグループ解析報告の注意点

　サブグループ解析の報告では，以下の点に注意する（表 9）．

① 事前に設定した仮説

　RCT などでは，患者の登録前から，サブグループ解析に関する仮説や計画がある場合もあれば，実施後に考案される場合もある．多くの観察研究でも，事後で

表 9　サブグループ解析報告の注意点

① 事前に仮説を設定
② 過去の研究で生物学的・病態生理学的に意味のある集団を解析
③ 全体の主解析で有意であった効果の解析が大原則
④ サブグループと治療効果に有意な交互作用があるかをチェック
⑤ 得られた知見は将来独立して評価

サブグループ解析が提案されることもある．少なくともサブグループ解析をする前の段階で，「臨床的に，〜の集団における…の影響について，われわれは興味があるため，サブグループ解析を実施する」と明言できるだけのロジックが必要である．

② 過去の研究で生物学的・病態生理学的に意味のある集団
サブグループ集団は，過去の研究で生物学的・病態生理学的に意味のある集団でなければならない．

③ 全体の主解析で有意であった効果の解析
全体の主解析で有意であった効果についてサブグループ解析を行うのが大原則である．少なくとも，それを意識して書く．全体の主解析で有意でなかったけれども，臨床的にこの集団の効果が重要である，というロジックが成立する場合に限り，そのようなサブグループ解析が探索的に行われることもある．

④ サブグループと治療効果に有意な交互作用があるかチェック
RCT などの仮説検証型の臨床研究で，サブグループによって主たる変数（介入など）の効果が異なることを主張するのであれば，サブグループ変数と主たる変数との交互作用を報告する．

⑤ 探索的であり，将来独立して評価
いずれにせよ，どのようなサブグループ解析も探索的であり，過剰評価はできない．サブグループ解析で得られた知見は，将来独立した集団で評価する必要がある．すなわちこのグループで効果があったのならば，将来このグループに対する独立した研究を組む必要があるということである．

(2) 多変量解析報告の注意点
多変量解析の報告では，以下の4点を必ず記載する（表10）．

① モデルの種類
時々，"multivariable regression analyses (model) …" と記載された論文を目にする．査読者は何のモデルかさっぱりわからないが，確かにわかることは「この著者は，多変量解析のことを理解せずに使っている」ことである．そのような論文に信頼性がおけるわけがない．

表10 多変量解析報告に記載すべき内容

① モデルの種類
② モデル選択の理由
③ 候補となる潜在的調整変数選択の理由
④ 最終モデルに導入された調整変数選択の理由

2章 論文の構成と書き方

② モデル選択の理由

多変量解析に使われるモデルはいろいろあり，それぞれに一長一短がある．多変量解析に使われたモデルをなぜ選んだかを意識する．多変量解析を記載するまでの解析内容によっては，モデルの種類を記載するだけでその選択理由が自明なこともあるが，少なくとも論文の執筆者はそれを意識し，ほかに選ぶ可能性のあるモデルがあるのであれば，今回の多変量解析で用いたモデルの選択理由を記載する．

③ 候補となる潜在的調整変数選択の理由

多変量解析は，単変量解析に交絡因子となる変数を調整因子として加えることとなる．この調整因子の加え方が恣意的であると，結果を恣意的に操作していることになる．調整変数を選択する前に，候補となる潜在的調整変数をどのようにして選択したのかを明示する．

④ 最終モデルに導入された調整変数選択の理由

多変量モデルを作成するのに「Stepwise法で導入した」と記載された論文をよく見かける．Stepwise法にもいろいろあり，Stepwise法以外の方法もいろいろあり，それぞれの調整変数選択法には，選ばれる理由がある．最終的にどのような理由・方法で調整因子を決定したのか記載する．必要があれば，複数のモデルを作成し，結果の堅牢性（robustness）を確認する．

2.6 Abstract（抄録）

Abstractは論文の要旨をまとめたものであり，論文では最も重要なパーツである．最初に編集者がAbstractを読んで査読に回すかどうか（即rejectするかどうか）を決め，査読に回すと決めたならば，どのような査読者が適切かを判断する．査読者もAbstractで論文の概要を判断し，本文の査読に取りかかる．PubMedなどの文献検索機関に登録されるのは，引用情報（論文誌名・巻・号・ページ）と著者名，タイトル以外にはAbstractだけである．多くの研究者は文献検索の際に，Abstractだけで論文の内容を判断する．また実際に掲載された論文誌においても，多くの研究者や臨床医はAbstractだけしか読まないことのほうが多い．

Abstractでは，実際に研究したことをアピールしなければならない．逆に一般的，総論的な議論や実際に研究したことと離れた結論が主張されると，編集者や査読者はrejectionに傾いていく．

2.6.1 キーワードをちりばめる

必ずAbstract中にキーワードをちりばめる．「前向き（prospective）」「ランダム化（randomized）」「横断研究（survey）」などのキーワードがすぐに目に入るような

記載を心がける．研究の特徴を示す重要なキーワードが Abstract に書かれていない論文は不利である．とにかく実際に研究を実施したことをアピールする姿勢が重要である．

2.6.2 具体的な数字を出す

Abstract の Results では具体的な数字を提示する．「X と Y に有意な相関が見られた」ではどれくらい関連するのかがわからない．「A 群の $X\%$ (n_1/m_1) の患者，B 群の $Y\%$ (n_2/m_2) に C が認められた（オッズ比 1.6 [95% 信頼区間 1.2-2.1]）」といった具体的な数字を出して実際に実施した研究結果がわかりやすい記述にするべきである．読者（編集者・査読者）は，具体的な効果や影響を知りたいのである．
- × "X was significantly associated with Y…"
- ○ "$X\%$ (n/m) of patients developed Y…"

2.6.3 Methods の分量 >> Conclusion の分量

Abstract の中でも Methods の分量を Conclusion より多く記述するようにする．Conclusion が 5 行もあるのに，Methods が 2 行しかなかったら，査読者は「何かあやしいぞ」と思う．Conclusion が 2 行で，Methods が 5 行くらいという分量が，査読者に「ちゃんとやっているなあ」という印象を与える．

2.7 Introduction（緒言）

　Abstract の後に引き続いて，Introduction を書く．
　Introduction とは，この研究を行おうとした背景である．また，この研究論文を理解するために必要な，基本となる情報，エビデンスである．査読者は，この論文を査読するに資する研究者が担っているが，必ずしも論文が扱っている内容に精通しているとは限らない．筆者のように方法論の専門家として査読することも多い．したがって，Introduction では，この論文で扱っているトピックについて，著者と同じレベルでそのトピックに精通しているわけではない，投稿しようとする論文誌の平均的な読者をイメージして記載する．逆に，医学生向けに説明するほどの基本的な事項から説明するのもマイナスである．

2.7.1 Discussion と整合性をもたせる

　次節の Discussion と整合性をもたせるために，Introduction は順番としてここで書くことになる．引用する際に，Discussion と同じ引用を使っても構わない（たとえば Introduction で引用した Reference 1 ～ 5 を，Discussion 中でまた引用してもよい）．基本的に，研究の背景となるようなデータの報告は Introduction で述べ，

著者が実施した研究結果と過去の研究(引用)を踏まえて，どのように臨床的に応用できるのかを考えるのであれば Discussion に入れる．

　　背景となるデータ　⇒　Introduction
　　臨床的な解釈　⇒　Discussion

2.7.2 書き出しが大事

　Introduction では書き出しも大事である．特に日本人の英文論文でよく見かける書き出しに，"It is well known…"がある．このような論文を山ほど目にする．Introduction の一番最初から It で始まるのは印象がよくなく，筆者は「It 症候群」と読んでいる．「この論文ではこれを扱うのだ！」という前向きな印象を最初に出してほしい．

　　×　It is well known…
　　○　Diuretics is…

　図 16 は 2 つの書き出しの違いを比較したものである．上の "With a paradigm shift in cardiology during the past few decades, the patient-centered practice has been widely acknowledged as crucial determinant of high-quality of care. …" は，何が言いたいのかさっぱりわからない．

With a paradigm shift in cardiology during the past few decades, the patient-centered practice has been widely acknowledged as crucial determinant of high-quality of care. Various studies have indicated that at least some elements of patient-centered practice have positive consequences on prognosis of patients as well as satisfaction and cost-effectiveness.[1-4]

Angiotensin-converting enzyme (ACE) inhibitors have been shown to improve the prognosis of patients with a variety of cardiovascular diseases, such as hypertension, myocardial infarction, and congestive heart failure, as well as diabetic nephropathy and other renal diseases.[1,2] As a result, the number of patients on ACE inhibitors has dramatically increased. In the United States alone, approximately 15 million prescriptions of lisinopril (the 11th most frequently prescribed medication) were issued for ambulatory patients in 2000.[3]

図 16　書き出しでは「この論文ではこういうことが言いたい」ということを述べる
(下：Morimoto T, et al：Development and validation of a clinical prediction rule for angiotensin-converting enzyme inhibitor-induced cough. J Gen Intern Med. 2004；19(6)：684-91)
(上：筆者の作成)

下の "Angiotensin-converting enzyme (ACE) inhibitors have been shown to improve the prognosis of patients with a variety of cardiovascular diseases, …" のように,「この論文ではこういうことが言いたい」ということを最初に書くことが大切である.

2.7.3 簡潔にまとめる

Introduction が長いと,Methods に読み進めるまでに疲れてしまう.冗長な Introduction は嫌われる.英文論文では A4 判用紙にダブルスペース(行間を倍に広げる)で 1 ページ以下が望ましい.4 ページも 5 ページも Introduction があると,大した研究をしていないと査読者に思われる.基本的には短く,スパッと「なぜこのような研究を実施したか」がすぐにわかるような Introduction を書く.

2.8 Discussion(考察)

Introduction に引き続いて,一気に Discussion を書き進めるのが,内容の不統一を防止できてよい方法である.

一般的には,表11 が Discussion で記載される内容であるが,必ずしもすべてをカバーする必要はない.基本的に,今回の研究のまとめや病態生理学的考察,他の研究との相違,臨床上における今回の研究の位置づけを Discussion で述べる.

過去の論文を引用する際に,無用に過去の論文の批判は行わないほうがよい.1 章でも述べたが,エビデンスとは,多くの研究者が,日々の小さな観察を,「科学的に」積み上げた共同作業の集積である(☞「1.1.1 論文執筆は臨床研究成功の最終作業」p.2).新しい研究が古い研究よりも何らかの点で優れているのは当然であり,過去の研究の礎があってこその新しい研究である.過去の研究で不備な点があったからこそ,新しい研究の意義が生まれたことを意識し,尊重すべきである.また,論文の査読者の多くは,その過去の論文の著者であることが多い.

表11 Discussion での記載事項

① 研究の主たる結果のまとめ
② 今回の結果の病態生理学的解釈
③ 過去に行われた研究(引用)との対比＊
④ 今回の研究が臨床に与える影響＊
⑤ 今回の研究の限界点・課題＊
⑥ 今後の研究の方向性
⑦ 結論

＊印は必須事項

2章 論文の構成と書き方

2.8.1 分量は Methods > Results > Discussion

論文の分量としては，多い順に Methods > Results > Discussion が理想である．Methods と Results を足した分量よりも Discussion の分量が多いということは，実際に行った研究よりも，著者の思いや他人の研究結果のまとめのほうが重要，ということになり，決してよい印象を与えない．

2.8.2 過去の研究と比較し，影響や解釈をまとめる

Discussion ではまず Results をまとめる．"We showed …" などで主たる結果を書き出して，その後に過去の論文と比較をする．総説論文ではないので，網羅的に論文を検索して，まとめなくてよい．研究や論文執筆の初心者は，頑張った自分の労力をすべて見せようとして，過去の論文を 20 も 30 も調べて全部 Discussion に入れたりする．せっかく調べたのだからと，すべてについて記載したくなるのはわかるが，読者（編集者や査読者）の視点からは，長いほど読み疲れるので，短くてよい．

特に，Discussion の分量を増やそうと，Results を繰り返したり，総説のように他人の研究を長く解説するのは印象が悪い．

研究結果をまとめ，過去の研究と比較した後，次のパラグラフで診療に与える影響や臨床上の解釈を行う．

2.8.3 Limitation（研究の限界）

研究の限界を述べることは必須である．Limitation のない論文はない．査読では「自分ができる範囲でベストの研究を行ったかどうか」が問われる．パーフェクトな論文というのは世の中には存在しない．「完璧でないことはわかっています．わかった上で，この環境で，このデータで自分はベストを尽くしました」ということを示すのが Limitation である．研究の限界を述べるだけではなく，その限界が結果の解釈にどのように影響するかを，簡潔に解説することも必要である．言い訳を書くのではなく，限界がどのように影響するのかを研究者が理解した上で，研究を実施し，報告するのが科学的な態度である．

2.8.4 Conclusion（結語）

Conclusion（結語）では，基本的には「自分のデータからのみ引き出す」ことが求められる．時々，Methods や Results とは関係なく「〜の患者を診るときには，…が重要である」と，著者の思いが語られることがある．Conclusion は思い（妄想）ではなく，Results から素直に引き出される事実である．もちろん，論文によっては，決定的な事実を打ち出せない論文も多いであろうが，その中でも，今回の研究をもとに「言えること」を主張するのである．

2.9 Reference（引用）

　引用を使ってよい場所は，Introduction，Methods，Discussion である．Reference が多いことは，決してよい評価にはつながらない．先述した通り，総説論文でなければ，文脈上必要な最小限の論文を適切に引用する．ただ一言の表現のために，論文をいくつも引用するのは無意味である．

- × Previous studies reported that substance X was associated with Y,[1,8]
- ◯ Previous studies reported that 45-65% of patients with substance X had symptom Y,[1,3]

　この論文をもとに，別の研究を孫引きしようとする研究者は，引用をもとに新たな論文を入手するが，編集者や査読者，ほとんどの読者はまず孫引きをしない．したがって，一言でよいので引用した論文からどのような情報を得ているのかを記載すると親切である．

　一般的に，臨床研究論文では原著を引用することを心がける．その他，教科書や報告書，近年では web page などから引用する論文を目にするが，学術研究は原著を媒体として積み重ねられてきたことを考え，できる限り原著から引用する．どうしても web から引用しなければならない場合は，web にアクセスした日付も記載する．

　引用にデータ（% など）ではなく誰かが何かを主張した文章（例 "Good writing is rewriting" — Truman Capote）は改変して引用記載してはいけない．引用句を使って原文に忠実に引用する．また，未発表論文や個人的な情報は引用としては原則避ける．

　英文誌に日本語の論文を引用することがあるかもしれない．和文誌でも英文の論文誌名を有していたり，Abstract が英文で提供されるものもある．そのような論文を引用する場合には，必ず引用論文リストに [in Japanese] と但し書をつけておく．海外の読者が勘違いして，日本語が読めないのに入手しようとしないためである．

　引用は，投稿しようとする論文誌の投稿規定に沿って作成する．ある論文誌に却下された後，別の論文誌に投稿することがあるが，この際に投稿規定，特に引用の記載方法を確認しなければならない．EndNote® などの reference software が使われることが多い．特に投稿する論文誌を変更する際に，いちいちフォーマットを手作業で書き換えなくても，自動的に投稿先に合わせた引用論文をフォーマットしてくれる．しかし，できあがった引用論文フォーマットはソフトウェアで管理された埋め込み文書状態になっており，別の環境で電子的にそれを開くと不都合があることがある．必ず投稿前には毎回コピー→テキストペーストでフォーマットを外す必要がある．

2.10 Acknowledgment（謝辞）

　一般的に Acknowledgment には，著者の基準は満たさないけれども，この研究（論文）に実質的な貢献をした研究者やアシスタントの個人名，場合によっては不特定多数の医療従事者や患者，組織などへの感謝の意を表したり，研究の実施に便宜を図ってくれた組織や研究費支援の情報を記載する．また，学会で先に報告した場合には，その情報を記載しておく．

　これらの情報をまとめて，論文の末尾に記載する（図17）．

2.11 Conflict of Interest（利益相反）

　Conflict of Interest（利益相反）とは，研究者（著者）が研究内容と関連して，他の組織と経済的，非経済的な利益関係を有するため，科学的な研究で必要とされる公正な判断が損なわれる「可能性」が存在することである．簡単に言えば，研究の結果，ある治療法が有効だと報告する場合，研究者やその所属組織がその治療法に関係する会社からなんらかの便宜を得ている場合，もしくは間接的に研究者にメリットがある可能性が疑われる状況である．これらは必ずしも金銭的なものに限らず，自己の昇進に関連する可能性がある状況や家族を介した利益も考えられる．Conflict of Interest は著者だけでなく査読者や編集者も，ライバル関係にある著者の論文の判断如何によっては，自分の業績や待遇が変わる可能性がある，など，広く「間接的」で「可能性があるもの」すべてが含まれると考える（表12）．

　ほとんどの論文誌では，論文を投稿する際にこれに関する情報を開示することを著者全員に求めており，その対象とする内容や期間は，論文誌によって異なるので，投稿前に確認して記載する．近年は論文とは別に，Conflict of Interest を別紙で提出させることも多く，論文誌の投稿規定に従う．

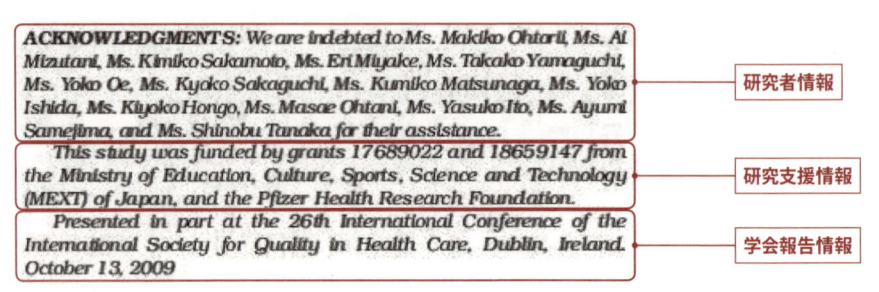

ACKNOWLEDGMENTS: We are indebted to Ms. Makiko Ohtorii, Ms. Ai Mizutani, Ms. Kimiko Sakamoto, Ms. Eri Miyake, Ms. Takako Yamaguchi, Ms. Yoko Oe, Ms. Kyoko Sakaguchi, Ms. Kumiko Matsunaga, Ms. Yoko Ishida, Ms. Kiyoko Hongo, Ms. Masae Ohtani, Ms. Yasuko Ito, Ms. Ayumi Samejima, and Ms. Shinobu Tanaka for their assistance. —— 研究者情報

This study was funded by grants 17689022 and 18659147 from the Ministry of Education, Culture, Sports, Science and Technology (MEXT) of Japan, and the Pfizer Health Research Foundation. —— 研究支援情報

Presented in part at the 26th International Conference of the International Society for Quality in Health Care, Dublin, Ireland. October 13, 2009 —— 学会報告情報

図17　Acknowledgment の例

（Morimoto T, et al：Incidence of adverse drug events and medication errors in Japan：the JADE study. J Gen Intern Med. 2011；26（2）：148-53）

表12　Conflict of Interest の対象となるものの例

1. 研究費
2. 相談料
3. 講演料
4. 原稿料
5. 旅費の提供
6. 委員会委員やコンサルタントなどの兼任
7. 雇用関係
8. 特許の保有や申請
9. 株式の保有

いずれについても，当該研究に直接関係ないものも含まれる．
(ICMJE http://www.icmje.org/coi_disclosure.pdf)

2.12 Title（表題）

　Title は論文執筆のどのステージで書いても構わない．論文の Title は，この論文を目にするすべての人（編集者，査読者，読者）が最初に読む部分であり，抄録の抄録として，一見して何についての論文であるかわからないといけない．そのような Title はすぐには思いつかないので，論文を書き進むなかで，思いついたものをメモしておくとよい．表13はそのような例であるが，一般的に総説的な Title は論文の内容を適切に示さないことが多く，注意を要する．また論文誌によって Title の字数制限があり，最終的にはその字数制限内で作成することになる．

表13　よい Title と悪い Title の例

- × Effect of beta blockers on cardiovascular events.
- ○ Lack of effect of oral beta-blocker therapy at discharge on long-term clinical outcomes of ST-segment elevation acute myocardial infarction after primary percutaneous coronary intervention.

- × Potentially inappropriate medication in Japanese elderly.
- ○ Epidemiology of potentially inappropriate medication use in elderly patients in Japanese acute care hospitals.

- × Current situation of treatment strategy for chronic total occlusion.
- ○ In-hospital outcomes of contemporary percutaneous coronary intervention in patients with chronic total occlusion.

- × Cost-effectiveness analysis of surgical treatment of pneumothorax.
- ○ Effects of timing of thoracoscopic surgery for primary spontaneous pneumothorax on prognosis and costs.

3章 文章構成

3.1 基本的な文章構成

　図18は，ある論文の実例である．標準的な分量で，仕上がり計6ページでまとめてある．

　そして，この6ページの中の，緒言（Introduction），方法（Methods），結果（Results），考察（Discussion）のそれぞれが示す部分は，図19の通り．分量の違

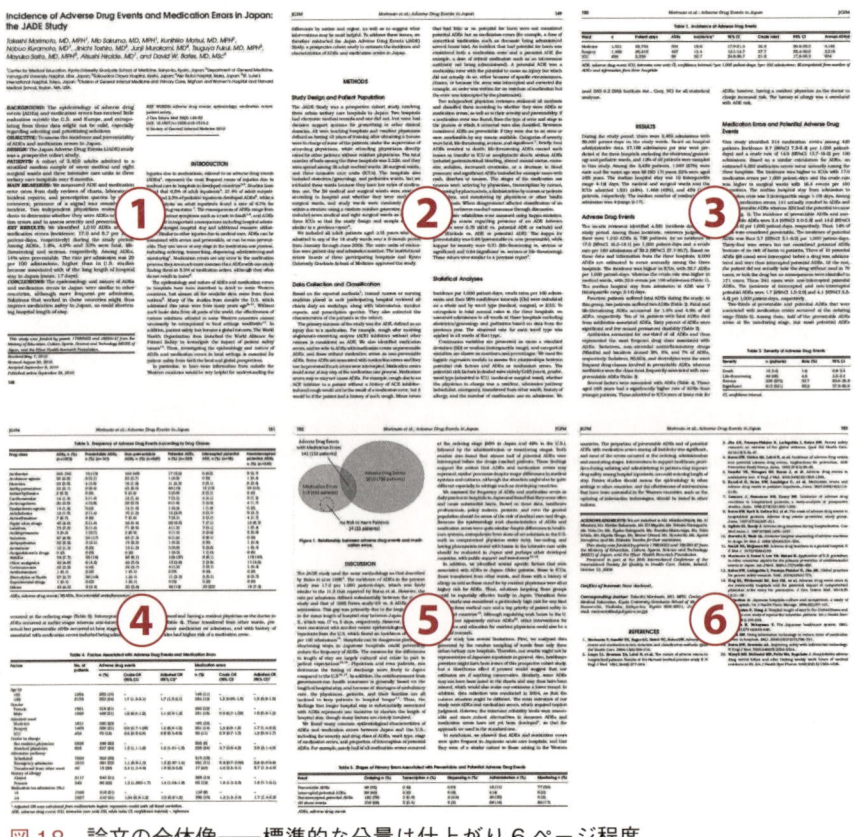

図18　論文の全体像——標準的な分量は仕上がり6ページ程度

3.1 基本的な文章構成

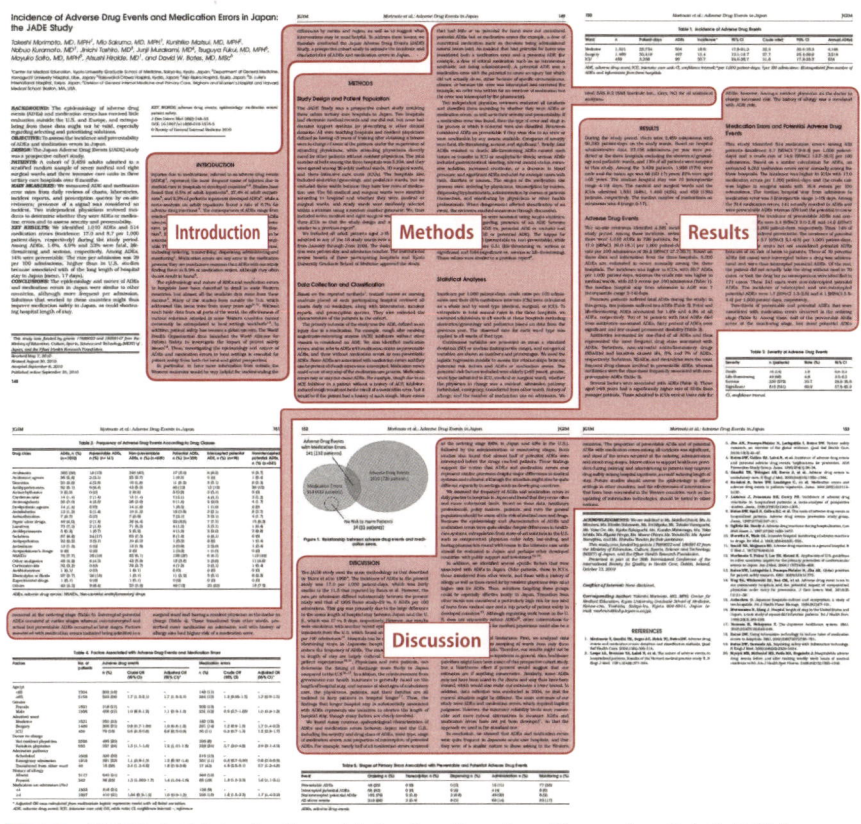

図 19 論文の中で Introduction, Methods, Results, Discussion の占める割合

表 14 投稿原稿で，各パートの占める割合（A4 サイズ，ダブルスペース，フォントサイズ 12 ポイント，標準的なマージン）

パート	ページ数
1. Title と著者情報	2
2. Abstract	2
3. Introduction	2
4. Methods	5
5. Results	4
6. Discussion	3
7. Acknowledgment	1
8. Conflict of Interest	1
9. References	3
10. Figure legend	1
11. Tables	7
12. Figure	1

41

3章　文章構成

いを見てとってほしい．この4つのバランスが崩れるとよい論文にはならない．
　この仕上がり6ページの論文は投稿時には図表含めて32ページ（ダブルスペース，フォントサイズ12ポイント，標準的なマージン）である．投稿時のページバランスは表14のようになっている．

3.2 センテンスとパラグラフ

　読みやすい英文論文とするには一つのセンテンスはできるだけ短く，また一つのパラグラフもできるだけ短くする．1パラグラフで，導入となる文章は1センテンス，本題は1～2センテンスでよい．さらに次のパラグラフへのつなぎは1センテンスで，論理的につながるように意識して書く．
　1パラグラフは図20くらいの長さにする．長くなるとよくない．読者（編集者・査読者）がリズムよく読み進められるように，シンプルな構造にするのがよい．

　① We assessed the frequency of ADEs and medication errors in daily practice in hospitals in Japan and found that they occur often and cause substantial harm. ② Based on these data, healthcare professionals, policy makers, patients, and even the general population should be aware of the risk of medical care and drugs.
　③ Because the epidemiology and characteristics of ADEs and medication errors were quite similar despite differences in healthcare systems, extrapolation from state-of-art solutions in the U.S. such as computerized physician order entry, bar-coding, and having pharmacists round with teams in the intensive care units should be evaluated in Japan and perhaps other developed countries, with public support and investment[18,19].
　In addition, we identified several specific factors that were associated with ADEs in Japan. Older patients, those in ICUs,

図20　理想的なパラグラフの分量（センテンスは①②③の3つ）
(Morimoto T, et al：Incidence of adverse drug events and medication errors in Japan：the JADE study. J Gen Intern Med. 2011；26 (2)：148-53)

3.3 日本人研究者の論文の特徴

　日本人が書く論文には，独特の特徴がある．以下に目につくところ14点を並べる．

① Titleと研究内容の不一致
　Titleに書いてあることと，実際に書かれてある研究内容が一致していない．原因には，先述したようにTitleがあまりにも漠然として総説的なTitleとなっている場合，もしくは結論と同じく研究結果ではなく，著者の思いがTitleとなって表

れている場合，である．
② 最初と最後の不一致
センテンスの初めと終わりが不一致な場合がある．また論文全体から見て，もっと広い範囲で Introduction と Discussion が一致していないということがある．
③ 冗長
先述したが，特に Introduction と Discussion に多く見られ，論文の全体の論旨から外れる総説的な内容で冗長となることが多い．逆に Methods は少々冗長と思われるぐらい，丁寧に記載するほうがよい．
④ 繰り返し
同じ内容のことを Introduction と Discussion で議論される．また Results で Table の内容を繰り返したり，Discussion で Results の大部分が再度提示される，などがある．
⑤ 定義していない用語が突然現れる
著者（研究者）にとっては，普段当たり前に使っている用語だと，何気なく記載してしまいがちだが，編集者や査読者，多くの読者にとっては何を指しているのかわからないことがある．略語に限らず，用語には常に注意を払う．
⑥ 同じものが場所によって違う単語で表現される
たとえば，被験者を指す用語が，最初は subjects と書かれていたのにもかかわらず，途中から patients という言葉に変わっている，ということはよく見かける．
⑦ 同じ用語が場所によって使われ方が違う
たとえば，control という用語が，最初は対照群の集団として使われていたのが，途中から対照群に投与される薬剤を指していることがある．⑥や⑦のような表現のズレは間違いなく査読者をイライラさせるため，投稿前にきちんと確認して直さなければならない．
⑧ 研究結果にないことが，突然主張されだす
2 章 Discussion の「Conclusion（結語）」でも述べたが，論文で主張するためには，根拠となる研究結果を，過去の他の研究者の研究の引用を踏まえて，論理的に主張しなければならない．論理的に結びつかない結論が Conclusion や Abstract でよく見かけられる．たとえば，ある疾患の患者の生活の質が悪いことを報告している論文で，Conclusion では「したがって，在宅看護師の充実が必要である」と結論づけているが，論文中では在宅看護師と生活の質との関連についてはなんら解析されていないような場合である．このような飛躍のある主張には常に気をつける．

・・・ここから先は英文論文に特徴的なものとなる・・・
⑨ パラレル構造の無視
英文には，常にパラレル構造がある．センテンスとしても，フレーズとしても，

単語としてもである．たとえば，Patients with hypertension, diabetic…という論文がよく見かけられるが，hypertension は名詞，diabetic は形容詞であり，本来並列できるものではない．フレーズでも，患者の特徴を示すフレーズと疾患の重症度を示すフレーズが患者採用基準の記載で or で並列して記載されていると，少なくともネイティブは奇異に感じる．

⑩ 主語に述語がない，述語に主語がない

頑張って英文を書いているのであるが，時々主語述語関係がわからないセンテンスを見かける．そもそも，このセンテンスの主語は何だろう？述語はどこにあるのか？と探さなければならないレベルですでにアウトである．こういう間違いを犯しやすい理由に，センテンスが長いことがある．日本語で考えた文書を英文に直す際，いろいろな形容句が間に挟まったりして，長くなるうちに主語の存在を忘れてしまう．したがって，できるだけセンテンスは短くして，単純な表現を繰り返すのがよい．我々は作家や詩人ではない．

⑪ 受動態が多い

受動態のほうが，能動態に比べて，センテンスが長くなる上に，自信がなさそうに受け取られる．後述するが（☞「3.5 英語の tips」右頁），たとえば，"All statistical analyses were conducted by using SAS 9.3 (SAS Institute Inc., Cary, NC)." とすれば，誰がやったかごまかせる．著者が自分たちできちんと実施したことに自信があれば，しっかりと We conducted と主語を明確にして述べるほうが，査読者としては安心して読める．

⑫ It や There で始まる文章が多い

2 章の「Introduction（緒言）」の項でも触れたが，It で始まる「It 症候群」（☞「2.7.2 書き出しが大事」p.34）のほか，There で始まる「There 症候群」も多い．主語が明確にならない上に，センテンスが長くなり，必ず受動態になり，査読者としてはストレートに読み進みにくい．

⑬ because と since

「～という理由から」という意味で since を使う著者が多いが，since には「いつからいつまで」という意味もある．論文の著者はきちんと区別して記載しているのだが，編集者や査読者は，しばらく読み進まないと，どちらの意味で使われているのかわからないことがある．場合によっては前に戻って読み直さなければならない．査読者や編集者に余計な手間をかけることはマイナスである．since はできるだけ避け，「理由」なら because，「時間」なら from を使うなどして，混乱を避ける．

⑭ 冒頭の although

パラグラフの最初から although と書き出す著者がいる．極端な例は，Introduction の最初から although である．「～であるが，しかし」と主題に入る前

の問題提起として使われているのであるが，印象としては「冒頭から言い訳？」と感じられる．but や however を文中に挟んで，問題提起から核心へ，と書き進めることは可能であり，最初からネガティブな表現を用いないほうがよい．

　これらの特徴が日本人研究者に多い原因として，アカデミックライティングを系統的に学ぶ機会が少ないことや，英文の原稿書きに慣れていないことがある．それ以外の原因としては，論文を書く際に，いろいろな過去の論文のフレーズを混ぜてコピー＆ペーストがよく行われていることもある．一昔前の，新聞の活字の切り抜きで作成した誘拐犯の脅迫状みたいなものを想像してほしい．その結果，上記で述べた②不一致や⑤定義されていない用語の出現，⑥同じ単語が違うものを指す，ようなことになる．また，論文執筆者や共著者による論文推敲が不十分なことも挙げられる．

　英文執筆に慣れていなくても，少なくとも自分で何度も推敲することや，共著者に論文を全面的に見てもらうことで，ある程度は改善できることであり，是非実施すべきである．

3.4　英語の掟

　論文の投稿規定を常に優先しなければならないが，英文論文においては，原則として記号はすべて半角にする．Table と Figure 内も同様である．日本人に多いエラーを表 15 に示した．

表 15　日本人に多い記号のエラー

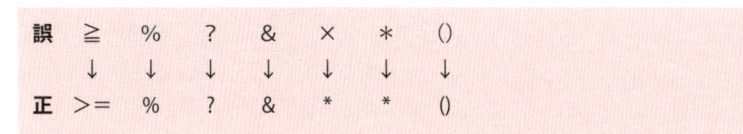

誤	≧	％	？	＆	×	＊	（）
	↓	↓	↓	↓	↓	↓	↓
正	>=	%	?	&	*	*	()

　数字，括弧，単位の前にはスペース 1 つ入れる．ピリオド，コロン，セミコロンの後にもスペースを 1 つ入れる．
　　Figure 1
　　Shown ()
　　155 kg　60 kg

3.5　英語の tips

3.5.1　能動態で表現する

　先に述べたようにできるだけ能動態で表現する．能動態だと文章が短く，自信

があるように見られる．
- × All statistical analyses were conducted by using SAS 9.3 (SAS Institute Inc., Cary, NC).
- ○ We conducted all statistical analyses by using SAS 9.3 (SAS Institute Inc., Cary, NC).

3.5.2 短い句で書く
短くできる句はできるだけ短く表現する．
- × in order to
- ○ to
- × conducted an investigation
- ○ investigated

3.5.3 大事なことは最後に
後に形容するような文をもってこない．センテンスで最も大事なことは最後に書く．後ろに because …などをつけないほうがよい．
- × We conducted a prospective cohort study of patients with diabetes because such patients are higher risk of deterioration of physical activity.
- ○ Because patients with diabetes are higher risk of deterioration of physical activity, we conducted a prospective cohort study of such patients.

4章 投稿と査読

4.1 Authorship（著者の資格）

　世界の主要医学雑誌の編集者の会議であるICMJE（International Committee of Medical Journal Editors：医学雑誌編集者国際委員会）が，著者の資格として必要な3つの条件を提唱している．ICMJEに加盟する主要論文誌はその会議の方針に従って，Conflict of Interestや著者資格などを共同で作成し，多くの論文誌はそれを踏襲している（http://www.icmje.org/）．それによると，原則として著者として資格があるのは，

1. 研究計画，データ収集，解析，解釈に実質的な貢献をした
2. 論文執筆作業への参加，論文内容の重要な点についての修正をした
3. 論文のResults，主張について社会的な共同責任をもつ

のすべてに当てはまる場合となっている．
　したがって，単に
- 研究費を取得した
- データ入手を行った
- 上司である
- 監督責任者である

というだけで，著者になれるわけではない．
　この条件に当てはめてみると，たとえば論文の捏造疑惑が出てきた際に，著者として名前が載っているのにもかかわらず「自分は関係ない」と責任逃れをすることはあり得ない．著者になったからには，内容について共同責任を負うというのが，この条件に入っている．
　Authorshipについては，誰がFirst Author（筆頭著者）になるか，という点も含めて研究開始前から意識しておくと後々スムーズである．できれば研究計画の最初に明確にしておきたい．
　First Authorは，基本的にその研究の実施，論文の作成に一番労力をさいた人である．多施設共同研究であれば，研究計画を作成し，施設を選定し，研究費を獲得し，データ収集をリードし，解析の方向性を考えた主任研究者やその代理人が担当するのが通常である．当然ながら，執筆の大部分を担当するのはFirst Authorである．2番目以降は，その論文の完成への貢献度の順番に並べる．臨床

研究では統計専門家が著者に入ることが多いが，解析や執筆，査読に対する対応への貢献度を考慮すると，当然2番目，3番目に位置されることになる．筆者も多くの臨床研究に統計専門家として参加しているが，authorの順番が後ろである研究（グループ）ほど，「貢献度は相対的に低いということですな」と解釈し，順番が前にある研究を優先して処理する．主任研究者はFirst Authorでなければ，Senior Authorとして著者リストの最後に位置されることが多い．

Corresponding Author（責任著者）は，論文執筆者を代表して論文についての対外的な窓口，代表責任者となる．論文の最終チェックから投稿，査読への対応，採用後の著者校正作業など，論文投稿に関するすべての作業を担う．投稿作業はアシスタントが代行するのも含めて，基本的にCorresponding Authorが自ら行う．

4.2 投稿先（ターゲットジャーナル）の決定

論文の主たるメッセージを届けたい読者ターゲットを考慮して，適切な論文誌を選択するところから始める．似たようなトピックで，研究対象やデザインが近い論文が多い論文誌は，最初の投稿先（ターゲットジャーナル）になりやすい．自分の論文で引用しようと集めた論文が最も多く掲載されていた論文誌はターゲットジャーナルになるはずである．

ターゲットジャーナルを決める際，教授クラスがFirst Authorなら時間をかけてじっくりと業績を狙ってもよいのだが，若い研究者が最高レベルと考えられるImpact Factorの高い論文誌（臨床研究ならN Engl J Med, Lancet, JAMAや，各領域のトップジャーナル）から順番にImpact Factorの低い論文誌に投稿するstep-down方式を行うのは，時間のロス以外の何ものでもないので，避けるべきである．もちろん，最高レベルの論文誌に「相当する」ような研究方法や結果である場合は，是非ともチャレンジすべきであるが，「相当する」かどうかは若手の研究者では判断は困難である．そこは主任研究者やCorresponding Author, Senior Authorの役割である．

ターゲットジャーナルが決まったら，その論文誌の投稿規定を徹底的にチェックする．

4.3 投稿の仕方

現在では多くの論文誌はweb siteを通じたonline投稿となっており，一部のローカルな論文誌のみメールや郵送での投稿となっている．投稿方法は論文誌の投稿規定に従って行えばよい．

ほとんどの論文誌ではcover letterを添付したり，online上でcover letterを直

4.3 投稿の仕方

接入力する場合がある．cover letter の書き方は研究者によって千差万別であるが，基本的に cover letter は査読者の目に入らない．唯一，編集者が目にするが，cover letter の内容如何で査読に出すかどうか，また採否を決めることはない．多種多様な cover letter や特に長い cover letter に辟易しているのか，cover letter のフォーマットまで用意している論文誌まで現れた（J Gen Intern Med http://www.jgimed.org/）．

　cover letter では，基本的に論文をその論文誌に投稿したい旨を述べ，一言だけ何についての論文かを説明し，投稿に必要な情報（研究費・先行発表）と Corresponding Author の連絡先を記載するので十分である．Abstract を繰り返して記載する必要はなく，まして Abstract 以上のことや，本文中にないこと（まれに見かける！）を記載するのはマイナスである．最初に述べたが，編集者は限られ

Xxxx（日付）

Dear XXXX
Editor-in-Chief,（論文誌名）

Title：（論文タイトル）

　Please find enclosed our manuscript entitled（論文タイトル）by (First Author) et al. We found that（主たる結果を一言で述べる）.
　This study was funded by grants from（研究費情報）．
　This manuscript has not been previously published and is not under consideration in the same or substantially similar form in any other peer-reviewed media. We presented an earlier version of the manuscript at the（学会発表を行っていれば学会名，場所，日付）. All authors listed have contributed sufficiently to the project to be included as authors, and all those who are qualified to be authors are listed in the author byline. To the best of our knowledge, no conflict of interest, financial or other, exists other than described in the manuscript.
　We would like hope that this manuscript is suitable for publication in（論文誌名）and we are looking forward to hearing from you.

Sincerely yours,

Takeshi Morimoto, MD, MPH, PhD
　（所属機関・住所・電話・FAX・email）

図21　cover letter の例

た時間でたくさんの投稿された論文を捌かなければならない．時間の無駄となることはやめてほしい．

　重要なのは，投稿しようとする論文を，過去に他誌で発表したり，他誌に投稿していないこと，学会発表歴があればその旨，すべての著者が著者の資格（先述）を満たすことを cover letter で宣言する．図 21 が cover letter の例である．

　投稿の際，査読してほしい研究者や査読してほしくない研究者（とその理由）を記載・入力することがある．査読してほしくない研究者については，その理由が妥当（ライバル関係にあるなど）であれば，まずその研究者に査読は回さない．一方で，査読してほしい研究者については，編集者としては，その査読してほしい研究者が著者とグルであり，不公平な査読をされると困るので，必ずしもそのとおりとはならない．特に著者とその推薦された研究者が近い関係ではないかと思われればその研究者にも回らない，と考えたほうがよい．論文誌や編集者はそうやって，潜在的な査読者情報を集めていると考えるとよい．

　投稿した後，そろそろ採否結果が返ってくるかな～と思っているタイミングになっても返ってこない場合，特に若手の研究者は気になるところである．忘れられてはいないか？アイデアが盗まれて誰か別のところで同じ研究がなされていないか？ライバルに査読が回って，嫌がらせされていないか？などである．

　論文誌によって，採否結果の初回報告までの日数はバラバラであるが，一般的に査読期間（査読者が依頼を受けて査読を回答する期間）は 2～3 週間である．査読者の査読の遅れや，編集部における前後の処理期間を踏まえると，1 か月半から 2 か月は問い合わせを控えたほうがよい．2 か月を過ぎた場合は，初回投稿時に与えられた論文番号を伝えて，丁寧に問い合わせを行ってもよい．一般的に，トップジャーナルほど採否結果の回答は早く，あまり有名ではない論文誌は，編集システムもきちんとしておらず，査読者のモチベーションも高くないので，3～4 か月待たせることも多い．

4.4　"Not acceptable for publication in its present form…" はチャンス！

　初回に採否結果が返ってきた場合，ほとんどの査読結果は "Not acceptable for publication in its present form…" である．これはチャンスととらえるべきである．point to point で論文を修正し，回答文書でコメントをつけて対応する．

　査読者の意見に納得いかなければどうするか？　反駁するのは，明らかに査読者が誤解している，間違えている場合である．それ以外の場合は，基本的に従うほうがよい．

4.5 "Statistical Reviewer" はビッグチャンス！

　トップジャーナルには，Statistical Reviewer がいて，解析手法の面に特化した査読がついてくる．Statistical Reviewer の査読がついてくるということは，編集者は採用を考えていることが前提であるので，これはビッグチャンスととらえてよい．基本的にすべての点について，Statistical Reviewer の指摘に従う．

　もし著者の研究チームに統計専門家がいる場合は，理由をもって査読意見の取捨選択ができる．時々，この段階になってから統計専門家に相談する著者がいる．このような状況は，裁判で，一審で敗れた後に慌てて弁護士を雇おうとするようなものである．統計専門家のスタイルはいろいろなので一概には言えないが，相手にされないことが往々にしてある．ちなみに筆者も相手にしない．本来は研究開始の段階から，遅くとも初稿を最初の投稿論文誌に提出する前に相談するのが原則である．

　Statistical Reviewer は研究の限界やいろいろな解析方法，オプションがあることをわかった上で著者を試している．完璧な研究などは存在せず，Limitation に書かれているように，限界があるのはわかっている（☞「2.8.3 Limitation（研究の限界）」p.36）．けれども，著者（研究者）はそれを理解してやっているのか，またはまったく理解しておらず単に統計解析ソフトを使ってポンと出した，たまたまの結果がこの論文なのか，ということを示してもらおうとしているのである．なので，きちんと答えれば採用される．

4.6 Rejection（却下）となったら

　泣く子と編集者には勝てない．たとえ査読者の無礼なコメントを目にしても，却下の理由が論文の曲解に基づくものであったとしても，決して怒ってはならない．無感情かつ冷静に，さっさとフォーマットを変えて他誌に投稿するのがベストである．何度も引用されるような優れた論文が，実はある雑誌で Rejection となったものであったということは，よくあることである．

　フォーマットを変えて再投稿する際に，却下された論文誌の査読意見が参考になれば，それに基づいて改訂する．全部言われた通りにしなくてよい．

4.7 Rejection だが姉妹誌に推薦されたら

　ここはチャンスである．たいていの場合，Impact Factor が下の（もしくはまだついていない）姉妹誌よりも，もっとよい論文誌に通ると思って他誌に投稿しても，うまくいかないことが多い．これも時間の無駄である．編集者は姉妹誌に掲載し

たいから推薦するのであり，きちんと査読意見に対応すれば，1回か2回で採択される．時間の節約は大きく，最終的にはよい論文誌に採択される．原則この誘いは受けるべきである．そもそも，姉妹誌をもつようなトップジャーナルは，仮に現時点では姉妹誌に Impact Factor がついていなくても，間違いなく数年以内に高い Impact Factor がつく．

4.8 査読者が困る論文

以下に該当する論文は，査読者を困らせるので，投稿直前まで，意識して確認する（表16）．

① 読みにくい論文

投稿規定に則っていない論文は，査読者をイラッとさせる．そして用語の使い方が不統一（先述）な論文も，査読者を困らせる．

さっきまで patients という単語が出てきていたのが，急になくなってあるところから subjects というのが出てきた．この subjects は，さっきの patients と同じなんだ！と気づくのに少し時間がかかる．使っている用語が不統一だとわかりにくい．

論文を書くときも，最近は，論文が電子化され，いろいろな論文をコピー&ペーストすることができるから，このパラグラフはあの論文から，こっちのパラグラフは別の論文からと，くっつけてちょっとまとめてしまうだけで，論文ぽいものができてしまう．すると，subjects や patients のように，同じ意味の異なった単語がばらばらに出てくることになる．

② 研究方法がわからない論文

本人はわかったつもりで書いているのだろうけれど，初めてその研究を見た人は，まったくわからないという論文は多い．省略せず，しかしくどくならないように丁寧に書く．

③ 長い論文

時間をかけて読むのは，査読者にとって苦痛以外の何ものでもない．

④ 結論が実際に行った研究から離れている論文

表16 査読者が困る論文

① 読みにくい論文
② 研究方法がわからない論文
③ 長い論文
④ 結論が実際に行った研究から離れている論文

この結論は，この研究からは成り立たない，という飛躍があってはならない．

4.9 書き方に関する論文の Rejection（却下）理由

論文の内容でなく，書き方によって，査読者もしくは編集者が却下する場合もある（表17）．

4.9.1 査読者からの却下理由
「いったい何が言いたいんだ？」と感じてしまう，メインメッセージがよくわからない場合は却下される．ほかに論文の構成が稚拙な場合，文章が稚拙な場合などは，査読者が却下する理由となる．

4.9.2 編集者からの却下理由
編集者は査読者に比べて，よりジャッジがロジカルでシンプルである．

スペースの関係もあり長すぎるものは載せたくないし，自己主張が強い論文も却下されやすい．文法やスペルミスは，編集者に発見されやすい（編集者はその道のプロである）．論文構成が稚拙という理由は査読者と同様であるが，Abstract が稚拙な場合も却下される．編集者は，Abstract をよく読んでいる証拠である．ほかに，revision（修正）段階のコミュニケーションがよくない場合も却下される．

これらの中のいくつかの理由で Rejection になる．

表17 査読者と編集者の却下理由

査読者	編集者
メインメッセージがよくわからない 論文構成が稚拙 文章が稚拙	長すぎる 自己主張が強い 文法やスペルミス 論文構成が稚拙 Abstract が稚拙 revision 段階でのコミュニケーション不良

第II部

論文 Before & After

　第II部では，実際に執筆された論文に対して，コメントを入れ，その論文が最終的にどのような形で掲載されたかを紹介する「論文Before & After」である．

　筆者が，未完成論文に対して，「雑誌に採用される論文」にするために，初回の修正点を容赦なく書き込んだ跡である．論文のどこに注目して，どう直し，最終的にどうなったかを見ていただきたい．

1編 不必要な言葉はいらない
同じ意味の言葉は続けない
用語は統一する

Before

Original Investigations

Epidemiology of potentially inappropriate medication use in elderly patients in Japanese acute care hospitals

Mio Sakuma, MD, MPH[1], Kunihiko Matsui, MD, MPH[2], Nobuo Kuramoto, MD[1], Susumu Seki, MS[1], David W Bates, MD, MS[3], and Takeshi Morimoto, MD, MPH[1]

[1] Center for Medical Education, Kyoto University Graduate School of Medicine, Kyoto, Japan
[2] Comprehensive Clinical Education, Training, and Development Center, Kumamoto University Hospital, Kumamoto, Japan
[3] Division of General Internal Medicine and Primary Care, Brigham and Women's Hospital and Harvard Medical School, Boston, MA

Author responsible for correspondence:
Takeshi Morimoto, MD, MPH
Center for Medical Education
Kyoto University Graduate School of Medicine
Konoe-cho, Yoshida, Sakyo-ku, Kyoto 606-8501, Japan
Telephone number: xxxx
Fax number: xxxx
E-mail address: xxxx

Presented in part at the 26th International Conference of the

International Society for Quality in Health Care, Dublin, Ireland. October 13, 2009

Word Count: 2,722 (Tables 4; Figure 1; References 22)

Abstract (250 words)

Background
Little evidence is available about the epidemiology of potentially inappropriate medication use among the elderly, which was proposed as Beers criteria, and the appropriateness of the criteria in Japan.

Methods
We conducted a prospective cohort study at random select wards of three acute care hospitals in Japan. Eligible patients were the elderly aged 65 years or older admitting these wards during study period. Trained research nurses followed the patients, and collected the data on medications and all potential incidents. Two independent reviewers evaluated all collected data. Updated Beers criteria were used to identify the use of potentially inappropriate medications and its effects on the patients.

Results
A total of 2155 elderly patients were eligible and 56.1% of them received at least 1 drug listed on the Beers criteria (BL drug). The rates of the BL drug prescriptions were 103.8 per 100 admissions and 53.7 per 1000 patient-days, and incidence rate of the BL drug related adverse drug events (ADEs) was 1.7 per 100 BL drug prescriptions. Compared those who received the BL prescriptions with those did not, older patients (P=0.0002) and those with more complications (P<0.0001) were less likely to have the BL drug prescriptions.

Conclusions
BL drugs were commonly prescribed for Japanese elderly inpatients, however, BL drugs related ADEs seemed infrequent. Our findings suggested that revaluation and further discussion will be crucial to consider usefulness and appropriateness of the Beers criteria before its application to Japan or other countries though it has been widely used in the US.

Introduction

Adverse drug events (ADEs) has been an important medical issue because they resulted in 3-7 % of all hospital admissions and were associated with a substantial increase in morbidity and mortality.(1-3) Elderly patients are particularly vulnerable to drug related events because of multiple co-morbidities and increased number of drugs taken. Therefore, the quality of medication use, especially use of potentially inappropriate medications for elderly patients is a serious public health concern.

In the US, to recommend avoiding medications with a high potential for adverse events and prefer alternatives with lower risk, the explicit Beers criteria were developed by the panels of expert geriatricians and pharmacologists in 1991 (4) and updated twice.(5-7) Since Beers et al. initially published these criteria, it has drawn considerable attentions and has been widely used to evaluate the qualities of medication use among the elderly in various settings.(8 -15)

In Japan, no similar criteria have been developed. Howeveappropriate medication use without any evidence of its validity among Japanese elderly. Applying the Beers criteria into Japan, it is crucial to clarify the epidemiology of the drug prescriptions listed on the Beers criteria (the BL drug) and their effects on health in Japanese elderly like other guideline developed outside Japan were not applicable in Japan.(16)

Thus, we scrutinized the epidemiology of the BL drug prescriptions among Japanese elderly inpatients based on the cohort of Japan Adverse Drug Events (JADE) study. We also investigated the BL related ADEs and the relationship between patients and doctors factors and the BL drug prescriptions.

Methods

Study design and patient population

JADE study is a prospective cohort study at three teaching hospitals in Japan. The total beds among three hospitals were 2224, and there were 26 adult medical wards, 30 surgical wards, and 3 intensive care units (ICUs) except the wards of obstetrics, gynecology and pediatrics. Obstetrics, gynecology and pediatrics wards were excluded and all 3 ICUs were included because the JADE study was designed to have similar study design and sample sized to previous report.(3) Fifty-six medical and surgical wards were stratified by hospital and whether medical or surgical wards. Then, the study wards were selected randomly within a stratum using random number generator. Thus, study wards included 7 medical wards, 8 surgical wards and 3 ICUs. The patients included in the JADE study were all adults aged 15 years or older, who admitted to any of 18 study wards over 6 month periods from January through June 2004. This study was approved by the institutional review boards of three participating hospitals and Kyoto University Graduate School of Medicine. Among the enrolled patients, this study included those aged 65 years or older.

Data collection and classification

Present report is limited to drug-related incidents occurring in people aged 65 years or older inpatients, and the primary outcome is ADEs caused by BL drugs.

We used the updated Beers criteria in present study,(7) which was initially developed in 1991 (4) and updated twice to reflect newly attained evidence on efficacy and safety of various medications.(5-7) Updated Beers criteria defined inappropriate medication use in 2 settings; 28 medications or classes of medications describing the potentially inappropriate use of medication applied to all general populations of the elderly and 35 drugs or categories of drugs that are inappropriate in persons with any of 15 known medical conditions.(5-7)

The definitions of ADEs, medication errors and potential ADEs were followed to previously clarified definitions (17): ADE is defined as injury due to a medication and may or may not result from medication errors. Medication error is defined as an error which occurs at any step of the medication use process such as drug ordering, transcribing, dispensing, administering, or monitoring. Potential ADE is a medication error with the potential to cause an injury but that does not actually cause any injury, either because of specific circumstances or chance, or because the error is intercepted or corrected. In present study, a few potential ADEs were considered as non error related potential ADEs because they had risks for injuries but not associated with errors.

The methodology used in present study was based on the methodology in previous reports.(3,17) First, one physician trained nurses and nurse students in an identical manner and placed them in each participating hospital. There, well trained research nurses collected all patients' characteristics as well as potential incidents, which included ADEs, medication errors, potential ADEs and others, reviewing practice data such as charts, laboratories, prescription data, reconciliations from pharmacy and incidents reports. They also assessed whether the BL drug was prescribed and its details if prescribed: a drug name, a dosage and frequency, the total number of prescriptions, instruction process, whether they were administered or intercepted, and who intercepted it if intercepted. Patients' co-morbidity was quantified using the Charlson co-morbidity index.

Next, two independent physician reviewers evaluated all collected data and classified all potential incidents into ADEs, medication errors and possible ADEs. When physician reviewers evaluated a possible incident as non drug-related incident, this incident was excluded. Furthermore, they categorized these incidents according to the following criteria: preventability, severity and the type of error and the stage in the process at which the error occurred if a medication error was present. ADEs were considered as preventable when they were due to an error. Severity was categorized into fatal, life-threatening, serious and significant according to the severity of incidents. When there were disagreement that affected classification of an event, reviewers discussed thoroughly and reached consensus.

Statistical Analysis

The unit of analysis was both the patients and events. Incidences per 1000 patient-days and crude rates per 100 admissions were calculated as a whole and by whether or not patients had any experience of receiving the BL drug prescriptions.

Continuous variables were presented with mean +/- standard deviation (SD) or median with interquartile range, and categorical variables were presented with number and percentage. To assess the relationship between patients characteristic and ADEs, we used t-test or Wilcoxon rank sum test when a patient characteristic was a continuous variable and Chi-square test when a patient characteristic was a categorical variable. The potential characteristics included were age category divided by 5, gender, admitted ward (medical ward, surgical ward, ICU), whether doctor in charge was resident (trained less than 3 years after obtaining licenses), whether operation was scheduled, sum of prescription categories on admission and the total number of complications on admission.

Results

During the study period, 2155 patients with 41649 patient-days were enrolled, and on-site reviewers identified 4019 potential drug related events, of which 13.1 % were not characterized as drug related events by the physician reviewers. Thus, 3493 potential drug related incidents were included (Figure). The mean (SD) age of these 2155 patients was 76.9 (7.6) years old and the most common age group was those aged 75 to 79 years (24.9%) followed by those aged 70 to 74 (24.5%) (Table1). Men (53%) were included more than women. 48 % of the patients admitted at medical wards, 40% at surgical wards and 13% at ICUs, respectively.

Among these 2155 patients, 1209 (56.1%) patients were prescribed at least 1 BL drug; 550 patients (45.5%) filled prescriptions for a single BL drug, 396 patients (32.8%) filled prescriptions for 2 different drugs of concern, and 263 patients (21.8%) filled prescriptions for 3 or more different BL drugs.

Compared these 1209 patients who received the BL drugs (BL group) with patients those who did not receive the BL drugs (946 patients, non BL group), patient and physician characteristics were both associated with whether a patient received the BL drugs prescriptions (Table 1). Older patients (P=0.0002) and patients with more complications (P<0.0001) were less likely to receive the BL drug prescriptions. In particular, patients aged 80 years and older had lower risk to be prescribed the BL drugs than those who were younger than 80 years (P<0.0001). There was no significant difference about sex between BL group and non BL group. In terms of physician characteristics, attending physicians are more likely to prescribe the BL drugs than residents (P=0.02). Doctors working at surgical wards prescribed the BL drugs more than doctors working at medical wards (P<0.0001). In addition, patients who had operation during hospitalization received more BL drug prescriptions than patients who had no operation (P<0.0001). Regarding the total number of categories of prescription that patients received on admission to hospital, significant difference was not shown between BL group and non BL group.

The total number of the BL prescriptions to these 1209 patients was 2237. Thus, the rates of prescribed BL drugs were 103.8 per 100 admissions and 53.7 per 1000 patient-days. In terms of the detail of prescribed drugs, a small number of drugs are a large share of total prescriptions of the BL drugs (Table 2). The 4 drugs with the highest prescribing frequency were hydroxysine (39.7%), pentazocine (35.3%), diazepam (9.5%) and bisacodyl (6.4%). These 4 drugs alone accounted for 91% of the total prescriptions of the BL drugs. The median dosages of these 4 drugs are 25mg, 15mg, 5mg and 10mg, respectively. Of these 2237 BL drug prescriptions, 731 prescriptions (32.7%) was intercepted before the drug was given to patients, and the rest of 1506 prescriptions (67.3%) was administered to patients (Table 2). Most intercepted prescriptions were a dose of medicine to be taken only once prescribed in advance in case patients requested it (94.8%).

Among these 1506 prescriptions which were administered to patients, we found 37 ADEs with 36 patients because two adverse drug events were counted for one patient. Thus, the rates of ADEs caused by the BL drugs were 2.5 per 100 BL drug administrations and 1.7 per 100 BL drug prescriptions. These 37 ADEs were associated with 11 different BL drugs (Table 3). Diazepam accounted for 9 (24.3%) of all beers drug related ADEs, and bisacodyl, hydroxyzine and pentazocine accounted for 5 (13.5 %) respectively. In terms of the manner of prescriptions order, the written order was the most frequent (78.4%) and verbal order accounted for 16.2%.

The most common ADE symptom was central nervous system symptoms, which accounted for 21 (56.8%), followed by gastrointestinal symptoms (24.3%). Severity of these ADEs was also assessed; no patient died of an ADE. The 5 life-threatening ADEs (13.5%) included 2 respiratory failures, 2 loss of consciousness and 1 hypotension. Furthermore, 22 serious ADEs (59.5%) and 10 significant ADEs (27.0%) were identified, respectively.

Comment

We found that prescriptions of the BL drugs were very common for elderly people aged 65 years or older in Japan.＊ Since Beers et al published criteria for determining the appropriateness of medication use in nursing home residents,(4) the criteria have been applied in various settings such as ambulatory care,(9) outpatient,(10) nursing home,(11) (12) or community dwellings (13-15) to evaluate the drug prescriptions in elderly population. However, there are a few small studies reported about the BL drug prescriptions for inpatients.(18-21)

Compared with these limited reports using different methodologies and in different population, the rate of the BL drug prescriptions in Japan seems almost similar to those reported in the US (18) and relatively higher than those reported in European countries.(19,20) On the other hand, the incidence of the BL drug related ADEs in Japan is lower compared with those reported in other countries.(19,20) These findings suggested that the frequent prescribing of the BL drugs had not been directly associated with increasing the incidence of ADEs in Japanese elderly inpatients. We should consider whether the Beers criteria are useful for avoiding the risk of ADEs in Japanese elderly inpatients is still unknown.

> この解釈を左頁の＊へ加える.

Several possible factors may account for the low incidence of the BL drug related ADEs in Japan. Japanese doctors' prescribing behaviors found in this study and common dosage of each drug, however, would partly explain it. First, common dosages of the BL drugs prescribed in Japan were different from those commonly used in the US. The usual dosages of the most commonly prescribed BL drugs such as hydroxyzine, pentazocine, and diazepam in the US are 50-100mg, 30-60mg, and 5-10mg respectively.(22) Compared with them, usual dosages prescribed in Japan are lower (Table 2). Thus, the common use of these lower dosages would protectively affect the occurrence of ADEs in Japanese elderly patients. Second, regarding to prescribing behaviors, the finding that relatively younger and healthier inpatients are more likely to receive the BL drug prescriptions suggests the possibilities that doctors subconsciously take care to avoid prescribing the BL drugs to the frail elderly. If more BL drugs were administered to frail elderly, ADE incidents might increase.

> これも引き続く文を読めば自明なので冗長.

We also found that attending physicians were likely to prescribe the BL drugs more than residents and surgeons than internists. These prescribing behaviours would reflect that they prescribe the custom drugs based on their experiences. Attending physicians are used to prescribing the BL drugs without awareness of their risks although there are appropriate alternatives for the elderly. Surgeons are also used to prescribing particularly certain type of the BL drugs such as pentazocine as their custom. In fact, pentazocine is one of the most frequently prescribed drugs while it is one of the most intercepted drugs (41.3%) (Table2). The main reason of interception of pentazocine was that patients did not request it though doctors prescribed it

1編 不必要な言葉はいらない／同じ意味の言葉は続けない／用語は統一する

beforehand in case patients asked it for relief of pain. The high prevalence of the interception of the BL drugs (32.3%) would be partly because of these prescribing behaviors: that means there could be many unnecessary medication uses for elderly inpatients in Japan. It would be a noteworthy finding in present study and should be one of the most concerned issues which need further investigation.

The present study has several limitations. First, it included only three teaching hospitals, therefore, the results may not be generalizable. Second, a bias might have decreased the number of events identified because the selected units were aware of the study and actively involved in it. However, unit sampling was required because our case identification strategy was too intensive and thus expensive to include all units. Third, another limitation is our event identifying system. We relied on record review and incident reports to find events. Therefore, events that either were not recorded in the chart or were not reported to us could not be identified. Because of these limitation factors, our rates would represent lower bounds.

Despite these limitations above, there are several advantages in present study. First, this is a prospective cohort study. Therefore, we can find the events caused by the BL drug prescriptions and assess the detail of them unlike other cross sectional study using national surveillance data. Second, present study was conducted following to the currently state-of-art methods.(3, 17) Thus, it will enable us to compare our data with other data reported using the same methodology and to consider about the differences of patient safety systems or health care management in each country. Applying the criteria or guidelines developed in other countries into another country in particular, the strict and appropriate evaluation using such a comparable data should be essential.(16)

＊

In conclusions, BL drugs were commonly prescribed for elderly inpatients while the BL drug related ADEs were infrequent in Japan, suggesting that the commonly prescribed BL drugs have not been directly related with increasing ADEs in Japanese elderly inpatients. Furthermore, we found there were several unique prescription behaviours among Japanese doctors and some of them would be related to unnecessary medication uses for elderly patients in Japan. Taking into account these findings, the current most concerned issue to improve the "appropriate" prescribing

---

generalizability はすべての論文についてそうであり，必ずしも limitation にならない．またこの1センテンスだけではどういう影響かわからないので，パラグラフを分けて詳細に書く．

Limitation には言い訳だけを書くのではない．その影響についての考察が必要である．

＊この部分にこの論文の結果の臨床への貢献を入れる．

for elderly would be the high prevalence of unnecessary medication uses rather than frequent uses of the BL drugs. Thus, further research and discussion and efforts for reducing unnecessary medication uses should be crucial before the application of Beers criteria into Japan.

無意味な使い方. discussion は当然である.

Acknowledgements

We are indebted to Dr. Jinichi Toshiro, Dr. Junji Murakami, Dr. Tsuguya Fukui, Dr. Mayuko Saito, Dr. Atsushi Hiraide, Ms. Makiko Ohtorii, Ms. Ai Mizutani, Ms. Kimiko Sakamoto, Ms. Eri Miyake, Ms. Takako Yamaguchi, Ms. Yoko Oe, Ms. Kyoko Sakaguchi, Ms. Kumiko Matsunaga, Ms. Yoko Ishida, Ms. Kiyoko Hongo, Ms. Masae Otani, Ms. Yasuko Ito, Ms. Ayumi Samejima, and Shinobu Tanaka for their assistance.

This research was funded by grants 17689022 and 18659147 from the Ministry of Education, Culture, Sports, Science and Technology (MEXT) of Japan, and the Pfizer Health Research Foundation.

References （省略）

Figure. Flowchart of patients

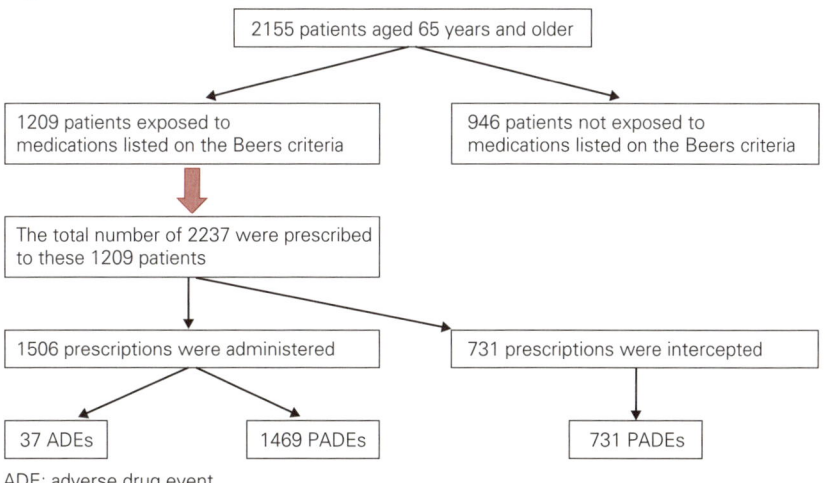

```
           2155 patients aged 65 years and older
          /                                      \
1209 patients exposed to              946 patients not exposed to
medications listed on the Beers       medications listed on the Beers
criteria                              criteria
   |
The total number of 2237 were prescribed
to these 1209 patients
   |
   +-----------------------------+
   |                             |
1506 prescriptions were      731 prescriptions were intercepted
administered                     |
   |                             |
   +----------+              731 PADEs
   |          |
37 ADEs   1469 PADEs
```

ADE: adverse drug event
PADE: potential adverse drug event

1編 不必要な言葉はいらない／同じ意味の言葉は続けない／用語は統一する

Table 1. Patients backgrounds, and its comparison between those who were prescribed the Beers drugs and those who were not.

Characteristics	Total No, (%) (N=2155)	BL drugs No, (%) (N=1209)	Non BL drugs No, (%) (N=946)	P value
Age group				
65-69　単位を入れる.	383 (17.8)	226 (18.7)	157 (16.6)	
70-74	528 (24.5)	311 (25.7)	217 (22.9)	
75-79	537 (24.9)	325 (269)	212 (22.4)	0.002
80-84	342(15.9)	177 (14.6)	165 (17.4)	
85-90	223 (10.4)	108 (8.9)	115 (12.2)	
≧90	142 (6.6)	162 (5.1)	80 (8.4)	
Hospitalized days, median (25, 75%)	11 (5,12)	13 (6,28)	9 (3,17)	<0.0001
Sex (Male)	1145 (53.1)	635 (52.6)	509 (53.8)	0.6
Race (Japanese)	2141 (99)	1202 (99.4)	939 (99.3)	0.6
Wards				
Surgical	854 (39.6)	590 (44.8)	264 (27.9)	
Medical	1025 (47.6)	479 (39.6)	546 (57.7)	<0.0001
ICUs	276 (12.8)	140 (11.6)	136 (14.4)	
Doctors in charge (Resident)	600 (27.8)	313 (25.9)	287 (30.3)	0.02
Operation (Scheduled)	511 (23.7)	413 (34.2)	98 (10.4)	<0.0001
The total number of categories of prescription on admission, median (25, 75%)	4 (3, 6)	4 (2.5, 6)	4 (3, 6)	0.4
Sum of Charlson score listed co-morbidity index, mean (SD)	2.1 (1.5)	2.0 (1.5)	2.22 (1.6)	<0.0001

BL: Beers listed
ADE: adverse drug even
ICU: intensive care unit

合併症の個数を表現するのに平均は不適当．しかし中央値（25％,75％）にすると，有意差はあるが表現上の差はなくなった．

Table2. The detail of Beers drugs prescribed during study period.

Beers Drugs	Total number of prescriptions	Dose/day median (quartile)	mean (SD)	Administered	Intercepted (%)
Hydroxyzine	888	25 (25,25)	28.4 (12.2)	599	289 (32.5)
Pentazocine	789	15 (15,15)	16.8 (14.6)	463	326 (41.3)
Diazepam	213	5 (5, 5)	6.3 (6.3)	146	67 (31.5)
Bisacodyl	144	10 (10,10)	10.5 (2.8)	118	26 (18.1)
Ticlopidine	40	200 (200,200)	187.5 (60.7)	40	0 (0)
Nifedipine	40	5 (5, 5)	5 (0)	23	17 (42.5)
Chlorpheniramine	35	6 (4,10)	7.1 (3.6)	32	3 (8.6)
Disopyramide	20	125 (50, 300)	162.5 (111.1)	19	1 (5.0)
Doxazosin	16	1 (1,2)	1.6 (1.0)	16	0 (0)
Cimetidine	15	400 (200, 400)	373.3 (148.6)	15	0 (0)
Pentbarbital	11	50 (25,50)	263.8 (741.8)	11	0 (0)
Triazolam	8	0.5 (0.5,0.5)	0.56 (0.18)	7	1 (12.5)
Amitriptyline	6	25 (10, 42.5)	30 (26.1)	5	1 (16.7)
Diphenhydramine	4	50 (50,50)	50 (0)	4	0 (0)
Indometacin	2	25 (25, 25)	25 (0)	2	0 (0)
Naproxen	2	450 (300, 600)	450 (212.1)	2	0 (0)
Amiodarone	1	250 (250,250)	250 (-)	1	0 (0)
Cyproheptadine	1	12 (12,12)	12 (-)	1	0 (0)
Thioridazine	1	30 (30,30)	30 (-)	1	0 (0)
Thyroid	1	100 (100,100)	100 (-)	1	0 (0)

中断されたのか，単に不要だったのかを分ける．

1編　不必要な言葉はいらない／同じ意味の言葉は続けない／用語は統一する

Table3. The summary of the Beers drugs causing adverse drug events

The BL drug	Administered	Number of ADEs	Rate (ADE / Administered)
Hydroxyzine	599	5	0.8
Pentazocine	463	5	1.1
Diazepam	146	9	6.2
Bisacodyl	118	5	4.2
Ticlopidine	40	3	7.5
Chlorpheniramine	32	1	3.1
Nifedipine	23	1	4.3
Doxazosin	16	4	25.0
Cimetidine	15	1	6.7
Amitriptyline	5	2	40.0
Thioridazine	1	1	100.0

BL: Beers listed
ADE: adverse drug even

detail かどうかは見たら
わかるので不要．

Table4. The detail of the types adverse drug events

Type of ADEs	Total No. of ADEs
Bleeding	2
Central Nervous System	21
Allergic reaction	1
Liver disorder	2
Cardiovascular	1
Gastrointestinal	9
Respiratory	1
Total	37

ADE: adverse drug event
PADE: potential adverse drug event

２つ目の単語が大文字で始まるのと
そうでないのが混在．最終的には，
論文誌の編集者がフォーマットに合
わせて修正してくれるが，査読者の
見やすさを考慮して統一する．

68

ORIGINAL REPORT

Epidemiology of potentially inappropriate medication use in elderly patients in Japanese acute care hospitals

Mio Sakuma[1], Takeshi Morimoto[1]*, Kunihiko Matsui[2], Susumu Seki[1], Nobuo Kuramoto[1], Jinichi Toshiro[3], Junji Murakami[4], Tsuguya Fukui[5], Mayuko Saito[5], Atsushi Hiraide[1] and David W Bates[6]

[1]*Center for Medical Education, Kyoto University Graduate School of Medicine, Kyoto, Japan*
[2]*Department of General Medicine, Yamaguchi University Hospital, Ube, Japan*
[3]*Rakuwakai Otowa Hospital, Kyoto, Japan*
[4]*Aso Iizuka Hospital, Iizuka, Japan*
[5]*St. Luke's International Hospital, Tokyo, Japan*
[6]*Division of General Internal Medicine and Primary Care, Brigham and Women's Hospital and Harvard Medical School, Boston, MA, USA*

ABSTRACT

Purpose The elderly receive many medications which may have adverse effects. Little evidence is available about the epidemiology of potentially inappropriate medications being prescribed to the elderly in Japan as defined by the Beers criteria, or whether or not these medications result in harm when used in this population.
Methods We conducted a prospective cohort study of patients aged ≥65 years who were admitted to three acute care hospitals in Japan. Trained research nurses followed up patients from randomly selected wards and collected data about their medications and all potential adverse drug events (ADEs). Two independent reviewers evaluated all the data. The use of potentially inappropriate medications and their effects on patients were identified using the updated Beers criteria.
Results A total of 2155 elderly patients were eligible; 56.1% received at least one drug listed in the Beers criteria (BL drug). The rates of BL drug prescriptions were 103.8 per 100 admissions and 53.7 per 1000 patient-days, and the incidence rate of ADEs related to BL drugs was 1.7 per 100 BL drug prescriptions. Among patients aged ≥65 years, relatively younger patients ($p = 0.0002$) and those with less complications ($p = 0.04$) were likely to be prescribed BL drugs.
Conclusions Although BL drugs were frequently prescribed to elderly Japanese inpatients, the incidence of related ADEs appeared infrequent. These data suggest that re-evaluation of the appropriateness of the Beers criteria is needed before they are used in Japan and other nations to assess quality or for decision support. Copyright © 2011 John Wiley & Sons, Ltd.

KEY WORDS — adverse drug events; epidemiology; geriatrics; inappropriate medication use; medication; patient safety

Received 14 May 2010; Revised 27 December 2010; Accepted 29 December 2010

INTRODUCTION

Adverse drug events (ADEs) represent an important medical issue because they result in 3–7% of all hospital admissions and they are associated with a substantial increase in morbidity and mortality.[1–3] Elderly patients are particularly vulnerable to ADEs as they often have multiple comorbidities requiring treatment with drugs. Therefore, the quality of prescribed medications in this population, especially of potentially inappropriate medications, is a serious public health concern.

The explicit Beers criteria were developed in the U.S. by panels of expert geriatricians and pharmacologists in 1991 and they have been updated twice since.[4–6] They include recommendations for avoiding medications with a high potential for harm and regarding alternatives with lower risk. Since Beers *et al.* initially published these criteria, they have received considerable attention and they have been widely used to evaluate the quality of medication prescribed to the elderly in various settings.[7–14]

No such criteria have been developed in Japan, but several Japanese physicians have applied the Beers

*Correspondence to: T. Morimoto, Center for Medical Education, Kyoto University Graduate School of Medicine, Konoe-cho, Yoshida, Sakyo-ku, Kyoto 606-8501, Japan. E-mail: morimoto@kuhp.kyoto-u.ac.jp

Copyright © 2011 John Wiley & Sons, Ltd.

criteria to avoid prescribing inappropriate medication even though their validity among the Japanese elderly has not been assessed. We believe that before widely applying the Beers criteria in Japan, it would be useful to evaluate the epidemiology of use of the drugs listed in the criteria (BL drugs) and furthermore to assess their effects on health among elderly Japanese, because other guidelines that have been developed outside Japan have not necessarily been applicable in Japan.[15]

We, therefore, scrutinized the epidemiology of BL drug prescriptions among elderly Japanese inpatients based on the cohort of the Japan Adverse Drug Events (JADE) study. We also investigated BL-related ADEs and the relationships between patients and doctors and BL drug prescriptions as factors.

METHODS

Study design and patient population

The JADE study, a prospective cohort study, proceeded at three Japanese teaching hospitals with a total of 2224 beds in 26 adult medical wards, 30 surgical wards, and three intensive care units (ICUs) other than obstetrics, gynecology, and pediatric wards.[16] Obstetrics, gynecology, and pediatrics wards were excluded and all three ICUs were included because the JADE study was designed based on a previous study with a similar sample size.[3] Fifty-six medical and surgical wards were stratified by ward type and hospital. The study wards were randomly selected within each stratum using a random number generator. Thus, we studied seven medical wards, eight surgical wards, and three ICUs. The patients included in the JADE study were all adults aged ≥15 years who were admitted to any of the 18 study wards during the period from January through June 2004, and this study included patients aged ≥65 years. The institutional review boards of three participating hospitals and Kyoto University Graduate School of Medicine approved the study.

Data collection and classification

The present report is limited to BL drug prescriptions in inpatients aged ≥65 years. We used the updated Beers criteria that were initially developed in 1991 and updated twice to reflect newer evidence regarding the safety and efficacy of various medications.[4–6] The updated Beers criteria divided inappropriate medication use in the elderly into two classes: 48 medications or classes of medications that are potentially inappropriate for the general elderly population and drugs or categories of drugs that are inappropriate in persons with any one of 20 known medical conditions.[6]

The data collection method was based on that described in previous reports.[3,16,17] Investigators trained nurses and nursing students in the same manner and placed them in the participating hospitals where they reviewed practice data such as charts, laboratories, prescription data, reconciliations from pharmacies and incident reports, and assessed whether a BL drug was prescribed and if prescribed, its details including name, dosage, frequency, total number of prescriptions, instruction process, whether they were administered or intercepted and if intercepted, who was responsible. They also collected potential ADEs as well as all patients' characteristics. Comorbidity in the patients was quantified using the Charlson comorbidity index.[18]

Next, two independent physician reviewers evaluated all collected data and classified all potential ADEs as ADEs or excluded ADEs. When potential ADEs were related with BL drugs, they were counted as the BL drug-related ADEs. On the other hand, potential ADEs were excluded when considered to be non-BL drug-related. Furthermore, incidents were classified based on severity, which was categorized as fatal, life-threatening, serious, and significant.[17] Disagreements that affected classification of an event were resolved by the reviewers through discussion and consensus.

Statistical analysis

The units of analysis comprised patients and the number of BL drug prescriptions. The incidence of BL drug prescriptions per 1000 patient-days and crude rates per 100 admissions were calculated. Furthermore, the rates of BL drug-related ADEs were also calculated by whether or not a prescription was actually administered.

Continuous variables are presented as means ± standard deviation (SD) or as medians with interquartile range; categorical variables are presented as numbers and ratios (%). Relationships between patients' characteristic and BL drug use were assessed using a *t*-test or Wilcoxon rank sum test when a characteristic was a continuous variable and the χ^2 test when a characteristic was a categorical variable. The variables included were age category (5-year increments), gender, ward of admission (medical ward, surgical ward, ICU), whether the doctor in charge was a resident (trained for <3 years after obtaining a license), whether an operation was scheduled, the sum of prescription categories, and the total number of complications upon admission.

RESULTS

During the study period, 2155 patients with 41 649 patient-days were enrolled (Figure 1). The mean (SD) age of these 2155 patients was 76.9 (7.6) years and the most common ages were 75–79 (24.9%) years followed by 70–74 (24.5%) years (Table 1). Slightly more men than women (53% vs. 47%) were included and 48, 40, and 13% of the patients were admitted to medical wards, surgical wards, and ICUs, respectively.

Among these 2155 patients, 1209 (56.1%) were prescribed at least one BL drug (Figure 1): 550 (45.5%), 396 (32.8%), and 263 (21.8%) patients filled their prescriptions for a single BL drug, for two drugs of concern, and for three or more BL drugs, respectively.

A comparison of the 1209 patients who were prescribed BL drugs (BL group) with those who were not (946 patients, non-BL group) showed that patient and physician characteristics were both associated with whether or not a patient received BL drug prescriptions (Table 1). Relatively younger patients ($p=0.0002$) and those with less complications ($p=0.04$) were likely to receive BL drug prescriptions. In particular, the risk of being prescribed BL drugs was lower among patients aged ≥80 years than among those aged <80years ($p<0.0001$). The ratio of males to females did not significantly differ between the groups with and without BL. In terms of physician characteristics, attending physicians were more likely to prescribe BL drugs than residents ($p=0.02$). Doctors in surgical wards prescribed BL drugs more frequently than those in medical wards ($p<0.0001$). In addition, patients who underwent surgery during hospitalization received more BL drug prescriptions than those who did not ($p<0.0001$). The total number of categories of prescriptions that patients received on admission did not significantly differ between the BL and non-BL groups.

A total of 2237 BL drugs were prescribed to these 1209 patients (Figure 1). Thus, the rates of prescribed BL drugs were 103.8 per 100 admissions and 53.7 per 1000 patient-days. In terms of the details of prescribed BL drugs, only a few comprised the largest proportion of total prescriptions (Table 2). The prescribed frequencies of hydroxyzine (39.7%), pentazocine (35.3%), diazepam (9.5%), and bisacodyl (6.4%) were the highest (91%) of all BL drugs and the prescribed median dosages of these drugs were 25, 15, 5, and 10 mg, respectively (Table 2). Of these 2237 BL drug prescriptions, 720 (32.2%) were not administered to patients, 11 (0.5%) were intercepted before being administered to patients by doctors or pharmacists, and the remaining 1506 (67.3%) were administered (Figure 1). The 720 prescriptions were not intercepted but not actually taken by patients because such medications were prescribed for symptoms which did not happened to patients.

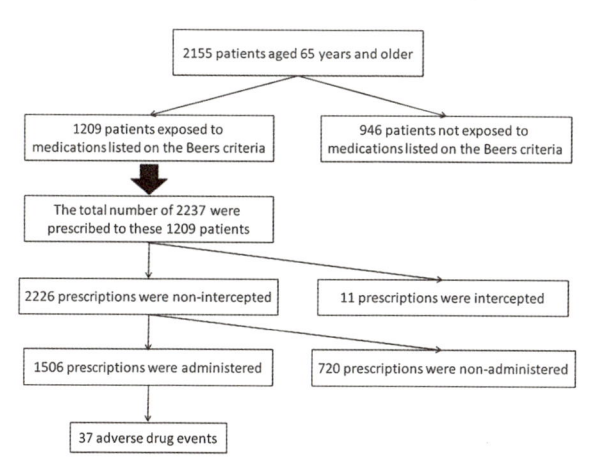

Figure 1. Flowchart of patients

Table 1. Patients' backgrounds, and comparison between those prescribed with and without Beers drugs

Characteristics	Total No (%) (n=2155)	BL drugs No (%) (n=1209)	Non-BL drugs No (%) (n=946)	p value
Age group (y)				
65–69	383 (17.8)	226 (18.7)	157 (16.6)	0.0002
70–74	528 (24.5)	311 (25.7)	217 (22.9)	
75–79	537 (24.9)	325 (26.9)	212 (22.4)	
80–84	342 (15.9)	177 (14.6)	165 (17.4)	
85–90	223 (10.3)	108 (8.9)	115 (12.2)	
≥90	142 (6.6)	62 (5.1)	80 (8.5)	
Hospitalized days, median (25, 75%)	11 (5, 22)	13 (6.5, 28)	9 (3, 17)	<0.0001
Sex (Male)	1145 (53.1)	636 (52.6)	509 (53.8)	0.6
Race (Asian; Japanese)	2141 (99.4)	1202 (99.4)	939 (99.3)	0.6
Ward				
Surgical	854 (39.6)	590 (48.8)	264 (27.9)	<0.0001
Medical	1025 (47.6)	479 (39.6)	546 (57.7)	
ICUs	276 (12.8)	140 (11.6)	136 (14.4)	
Doctor in charge (Resident)	600 (27.8)	313 (25.9)	287 (30.3)	0.02
Surgery (Scheduled)	511 (23.7)	413 (34.2)	98 (10.4)	<0.0001
Total number of categories of prescription on admission, median (25, 75%)	4 (3, 6)	4 (2.5, 6)	4 (3, 6)	0.4
Charlson comorbidity index, median (25, 75%).	3 (1, 5)	3 (1, 5)	3 (1, 5)	0.04

BL drugs, drugs listed in the Beers criteria; ADE, adverse drug event; ICU, intensive care unit.

Among the 1506 prescriptions that were administered to patients, we found that 37 ADEs occurred in 36 patients because one patient developed two events (Figure 1). Thus, the rates of ADEs caused by the BL drugs were 2.5 per 100 BL drug administrations and 1.7 per 100 BL drug prescriptions. These 37 ADEs were associated with 11 BL drugs (Table 3). Diazepam accounted for nine (24.3%) of all BL drug-related ADEs, and bisacodyl, hydroxyzine, and pentazocine accounted for five (13.5%) each (Table 3). Written orders for prescriptions were the most frequent (78.4%) among BL drug-related ADEs and verbal order accounted for 16.2%.

The most common category of symptoms associated with ADEs were central nervous system symptoms, which totaled 21 (56.8%), followed by gastrointestinal symptoms (24.3%) (Table 4). None of the patients died of an ADE. The five life-threatening ADEs (13.5%) were respiratory failure ($n=2$), loss of consciousness ($n=2$), and hypotension ($n=1$). All life-threatening

Table 2. Details of Beers drugs prescribed during the study period

BL drugs	Total prescriptions	Dose/day median (quartile)	Mean (SD)	Administered	Intercepted (%)	Not administered because of unnecessary (%)
Hydroxyzine	888	25 (25, 25)	28.4 (12.2)	599	7 (0.8)	282 (31.8)
Pentazocine	789	15 (15, 15)	16.8 (14.6)	463	0 (0)	326 (41.3)
Diazepam	213	5 (5, 5)	6.3 (6.3)	146	1 (0.5)	66 (31.0)
Bisacodyl	144	10 (10, 10)	10.5 (2.8)	118	2 (1.4)	24 (16.7)
Ticlopidine	40	200 (200, 200)	187.5 (60.7)	40	0 (0)	0 (0)
Nifedipine	40	5 (5, 5)	5 (0)	23	0 (0)	17 (42.5)
Chlorpheniramine	35	6 (4,10)	7.1 (3.6)	32	0 (0)	3 (8.6)
Disopyramide	20	125 (50, 300)	162.5 (111.1)	19	0 (0)	1 (5.0)
Doxazosin	16	1 (1,2)	1.6 (1.0)	16	0 (0)	0 (0)
Cimetidine	15	400 (200, 400)	373.3 (148.6)	15	0 (0)	0 (0)
Pentobarbital	11	50 (25, 50)	263.8 (741.8)	11	0 (0)	0 (0)
Triazolam	8	0.5 (0.5, 0.5)	0.56 (0.18)	7	1 (12.5)	0 (0)
Amitriptyline	6	25 (10, 42.5)	30 (26.1)	5	0 (0)	1 (16.7)
Diphenhydramine	4	50 (50, 50)	50 (0)	4	0 (0)	0 (0)
Indomethacin	2	25 (25, 25)	25 (0)	2	0 (0)	0 (0)
Naproxen	2	450 (300, 600)	450 (212.1)	2	0 (0)	0 (0)
Amiodarone	1	250 (250, 250)	250 (-)	1	0 (0)	0 (0)
Cyproheptadine	1	12 (12, 12)	12 (-)	1	0 (0)	0 (0)
Thioridazine	1	30 (30, 30)	30 (-)	1	0 (0)	0 (0)
Thyroid	1	100 (100, 100)	100 (-)	1	0 (0)	0 (0)

BL drugs, drugs listed in the Beers criteria.

Table 3. Summary of Beers drugs causing adverse drug events

BL drugs	Administered	Number of ADEs	Rate (ADE/Administered)
Hydroxyzine	599	5	0.8
Pentazocine	463	5	1.1
Diazepam	146	9	6.2
Bisacodyl	118	5	4.2
Ticlopidine	40	3	7.5
Chlorpheniramine	32	1	3.1
Nifedipine	23	1	4.3
Doxazosin	16	4	25.0
Cimetidine	15	1	6.7
Amitriptyline	5	2	40.0
Thioridazine	1	1	100.0

BL drugs, drugs listed in the Beers criteria; ADE, adverse drug event.

cases were caused by diazepam except for hypotension by pentazocine. We also identified 22 (59.5%) serious and 10 (27.9%) significant ADEs.

DISCUSSION

We found that patients aged 65 years or elder were frequently prescribed Beers List drugs in Japan, but the incidence of harm was quite low. Even among the ADEs which did occur, many were caused by diazepam, which should not be used in the elderly because there are a number of safer alternatives, and the rate for the remaining drugs was very low. These data suggest that the full Beers List may have limitations in Japan.

Since Beers *et al*. published criteria for determining the appropriateness of medication in nursing home residents, the criteria have been applied to evaluate drugs prescribed to the elderly in various settings, including ambulatory care,[12] outpatients,[13] nursing homes,[7,14] and community dwellings.[8,10,11]

Few studies have described BL drug prescriptions for inpatients (Table 5).[19–22] Compared with these reports using different methodologies and in different populations, the rate of BL drug prescriptions in Japan seems higher than those reported in the U.S. and in

Table 4. Types of adverse drug events

Types of ADEs	Total
Bleeding	2
Central nervous system	21
Allergic reaction	1
Liver disorder	2
Cardiovascular	1
Gastrointestinal	9
Respiratory	1
Total	37

ADE, adverse drug event.

Copyright © 2011 John Wiley & Sons, Ltd.

European countries (Table 5). There is no data on the incidence of ADEs due to BL drugs, and our study is the first report on inpatients setting. The incidence of the BL drug-related ADEs in Japan is relatively low considering high frequency of BL drug prescriptions. These findings suggested that the frequent prescription of BL drugs has not been directly associated with an increasing incidence of ADEs among elderly Japanese inpatients on acute care hospitals. Whether or not the Beers criteria as a group are in fact helpful for avoiding the risk of ADEs among this population remains questionable.

Several factors might account for the low incidence of the BL drug-related ADEs in Japan. The prescribing behaviors of Japanese physicians identified in this study and the common dosages of each drug might be partial explanations. The common dosages of BL drugs prescribed in Japan and in the U.S. differed. The usual dose ranges of the most commonly prescribed BL drugs, such as hydroxyzine, pentazocine, and diazepam in the U.S., are 50–100, 30–60, and 5–10 mg, respectively,[23] but these ranges are lower in Japan (Table 2). Thus, the application of lower dosages would protect against the occurrence of ADEs among elderly Japanese patients. Furthermore, such drugs are prescribed temporarily for some occasions such as premedication for operation or pain controls. Such temporal use of select BL drugs would also protect patients from the incidence of ADEs rather than long-term use of BL drugs in ambulatory settings.

The finding that relatively younger and healthier inpatients are more likely to be prescribed with BL drugs suggests that physicians may already avoid prescribing them to frail elderly patients. The incidence of ADEs might increase if more BL drugs were administered to this group of patients.

We also found that BL drugs were more likely to be prescribed by attending physicians than residents, and by surgeons than internists. These prescribing behaviors would reflect the habit of prescribing custom drugs based on experience. Attending physicians habitually prescribe BL drugs without awareness of their risks, although better alternatives for the elderly are often available. Surgeons also customarily prescribe certain specific types of BL drugs, such as pentazocine, which is one of the most frequently prescribed for pain, even though it had one of the highest frequencies of not being administered (in 41.3% of orders, it was not used). The main reason for this was simply that patients did not complain of pain. The high prevalence of these non-administered BL drug prescriptions (in 32.2% of all BL drug prescription, they were not used) could be partly

Pharmacoepidemiology and Drug Safety, 2011; **20**: 386–392
DOI: 10.1002/pds

Table 5. Comparison of the rate of Beers drug prescriptions and adverse drug events

Study	JADE study	Onder G	Egger S	Rothberg M	Corsonello A
Country	Japan	Italy	Switzerland	U.S.	Italy
Setting	Three acute teaching hospitals	Community and university hospitals	1 teaching hospital	384 small- to medium- sized non-teaching hospitals	Community and university hospitals
Wards	Seven medical wards/eight surgical wards/3 ICUs	81 geriatric and internal medicine wards	One general medical ward/One geriatric ward	Patients with seven selected diagnoses on all wards	11 acute care medical wards/three long-term care and rehabilitation units
Number of patients	2155	5152	800	493 971	506
Data acquisition method	Reviewers	Reviewers	Database	Database	Reviewers
No. of patients receiving BL drug/100 patients	56.1	28.6	16.0 (medical ward)/20.8 (geriatric ward)	49	20.6
No. of BL drug-related ADEs/100 BL drug administrations	2.5	Not available	Not available	Not available	Not available

BL drugs, drugs listed in the Beers criteria; ADE, adverse drug event; ICU, intensive care unit.

because of such prescription behaviors among Japanese physicians, which means that many unnecessary medications could be ordered to elderly inpatients in Japan. This is a notable finding of the present study that warrants further investigation.

We tried to obtain generalizable data by using random select wards from three acute teaching hospitals, but the results should be different in other settings such as nursing homes or outpatients. The low incidence of ADE related to BL drugs should be taken into account that the duration of medication use among inpatients on acute hospitals is relatively shorter than other settings. To scrutinize the safety profile of BL drugs, further research in different settings, such as outpatients, nursing homes, or community dwellings, are needed in Japan as well as worldwide.

This study has several limitations. Bias might have decreased or increased the number of events identified because the selected units were aware of the study and actively involved in it. However, if anything the physicians in the units would have been likely to prescribe more conservatively than they would have otherwise. Our event identification system has another limitation in that we relied on record review and incident reports to find ADEs. Therefore, we would have missed ADEs that were not recorded in charts or reported to us. These factors might have led to an underestimation of ADE rates.

The present study has several advantages despite these limitations. Since it was a prospective cohort study, events caused by BL drug prescriptions could be identified and detailed case assessments could be done, unlike in cross-sectional studies using national surveillance data. The study proceeded according to state-of-the-art methodology;[3,17] thus, our rates should be comparable to other findings done using the same methodology. This should in turn facilitate assessment of differences in patient safety systems and health care management in various countries. Before applying criteria or guidelines developed in one country to another, strict and appropriate evaluation of such comparable data is essential.[15] In the future, drugs will likely be ordered primarily through computerized physician order entry, and these applications can suggest both appropriate age-related dosages and avoiding certain medications which are truly high-risk in the elderly.[24]

In conclusion, BL drugs are frequently prescribed for elderly inpatients in Japan, whereas ADEs related to these drugs are infrequent, suggesting that commonly prescribed BL drugs have not been directly associated with increasing ADEs among this patient population. Furthermore, we found specific prescribing behaviors among Japanese physicians in particular with use of lower dosages, which may have decreased the risk of harm in elderly Japanese patients. Taking into account these findings, the most critical issue involved in improving "appropriate" prescription for the elderly appears to be the high prevalence of unnecessary medication rather than frequent use of BL drugs. Thus, further study and efforts to reduce unnecessary medication use are needed before applying the Beers criteria in Japan, especially as a tool for assessing the quality of prescribing across a population.

CONFLICT OF INTEREST

All authors listed have contributed sufficiently to the project to be included as authors, and all those who are qualified to be authors are listed in the author byline.

> **KEY POINTS**
> - More than half of elderly inpatients were prescribed potentially inappropriate medications in Japanese acute care hospitals.
> - Interception of such medication by healthcare providers was only 0.5%. ADEs occurred in 2.5% of those actually administered.

There was no potential conflict of interest other than description below: Dr David Bates is on the clinical advisory board for Patient Safety Systems, which provides a set of approaches to help hospitals improve safety. He consults for Hearst, which develops knowledge resources. He also serves on the clinical advisory board for SEA Medical Systems, which makes intravenous pump technology.

ACKNOWLEDGEMENTS

The authors are indebted to Ms Makiko Ohtorii, Ms Ai Mizutani, Ms Kimiko Sakamoto, Ms Eri Miyake, Ms Takako Yamaguchi, Ms Yoko Oe, Ms Kyoko Sakaguchi, Ms Kumiko Matsunaga, Ms Yoko Ishida, Ms Kiyoko Hongo, Ms Masae Otani, Ms Yasuko Ito, Ms Ayumi Samejima, and Ms Shinobu Tanaka for their assistance.

This study was funded by grants 17689022 and 18659147 from the Ministry of Education, Culture, Sports, Science and Technology (MEXT) of Japan, and the Pfizer Health Research Foundation. These funding sources had no role in design and conduct of the study; collection, management, analysis, and interpretation of the data; and preparation, review, or approval of the manuscript.

REFERENCES

1. Leape LL, Brennan TA, Laird N, et al. The nature of adverse events in hospitalized patients. Results of the Harvard Medical Practice Study II. N Engl J Med 1991; 324(6): 377–384.
2. Brennan TA, Leape LL, Laird NM, et al. Incidence of adverse events and negligence in hospitalized patients. Results of the Harvard Medical Practice Study I. N Engl J Med 1991; 324(6): 370–376.
3. Bates DW, Cullen DJ, Laird N, et al. Incidence of adverse drug events and potential adverse drug events. Implications for prevention. ADE Prevention Study Group. JAMA 1995; 274(1): 29–34.
4. Beers MH, Ouslander JG, Rollingher I, Reuben DB, Brooks J, Beck JC. Explicit criteria for determining inappropriate medication use in nursing home residents. UCLA Division of Geriatric Medicine. Arch Intern Med 1991; 151(9): 1825–1832.
5. Beers MH. Explicit criteria for determining potentially inappropriate medication use by the elderly. An update. Arch Intern Med 1997; 157(14): 1531–1536.
6. Fick DM, Cooper JW, Wade WE, Waller JL, Maclean JR, Beers MH. Updating the Beers criteria for potentially inappropriate medication use in older adults: results of a US consensus panel of experts. Arch Intern Med 2003; 163(22): 2716–2724.
7. Beers MH, Ouslander JG, Fingold SF, et al. Inappropriate medication prescribing in skilled-nursing facilities. Ann Intern Med 1992; 117(8): 684–689.
8. Stuck AE, Beers MH, Steiner A, Aronow HU, Rubenstein LZ, Beck JC. Inappropriate medication use in community-residing older persons. Arch Intern Med 1994; 154(19): 2195–2200.
9. Willcox SM, Himmelstein DU, Woolhandler S. Inappropriate drug prescribing for the community-dwelling elderly. JAMA 1994; 272(4): 292–296.
10. Zhan C, Sangl J, Bierman AS, et al. Potentially inappropriate medication use in the community-dwelling elderly: findings from the 1996; Medical Expenditure Panel Survey JAMA 2001; 286(22): 2823–2829.
11. Hanlon JT, Fillenbaum GG, Kuchibhatla M, et al. Impact of inappropriate drug use on mortality and functional status in representative community dwelling elders. Med Care 2002; 40(2): 166–176.
12. Goulding MR. Inappropriate medication prescribing for elderly ambulatory care patients. Arch Intern Med 2004; 164(3): 305–312.
13. Curtis LH, Ostbye T, Sendersky V, et al. Inappropriate prescribing for elderly Americans in a large outpatient population. Arch Intern Med 2004; 164(15): 1621–1625.
14. Fialova D, Topinkova E, Gambassi G, et al. Potentially inappropriate medication use among elderly home care patients in Europe. JAMA 2005; 293(11): 1348–1358.
15. Morimoto T, Fukui T, Lee TH, Matsui K. Application of U.S. guidelines in other countries: aspirin for the primary prevention of cardiovascular events in Japan. Am J Med 2004; 117(7): 459–468.
16. Morimoto T, Sakuma M, Matsui K, et al. Incidence of Adverse Drug Events and Medication Errors in Japan: the JADE Study. J Gen Intern Med 2011; 26(2): 148–153.
17. Morimoto T, Gandhi TK, Seger AC, Hsieh TC, Bates DW. Adverse drug events and medication errors: detection and classification methods. Qual Saf Health Care 2004; 13(4): 306–314.
18. Charlson ME, Pompei P, Ales KL, MacKenzie CR. A new method of classifying prognostic comorbidity in longitudinal studies: development and validation. J Chronic Dis 1987; 40(5): 373–383.
19. Onder G, Landi F, Liperoti R, Fialova D, Gambassi G, Bernabei R. Impact of inappropriate drug use among hospitalized older adults. Eur J Clin Pharmacol 2005; 61(5–6): 453–459.
20. Egger SS, Bachmann A, Hubmann N, Schlienger RG, Krahenbuhl S. Prevalence of potentially inappropriate medication use in elderly patients: comparison between general medical and geriatric wards. Drugs Aging 2006; 23(10): 823–837.
21. Rothberg MB, Pekow PS, Liu F, et al. Potentially inappropriate medication use in hospitalized elders. J Hosp Med 2008; 3(2): 91–102.
22. Corsonello A, Pedone C, Lattanzio F, et al. Potentially inappropriate medications and functional decline in elderly hospitalized patients. J Am Geriatr Soc 2009; 57(6): 1007–1014.
23. The Merck Manuals online medical library. http://www.merck.com/mmpe/index.html [19 April 2010].
24. Peterson JF, Kuperman GJ, Shek C, Patel M, Avorn J, Bates DW. Guided prescription of psychotropic medications for geriatric inpatients. Arch Intern Med 2005; 165(7): 802–807.

(Sakuma M, et al.：Epidemiology of potentially inappropriate medication use in elderly patients in Japanese acute care hospitals. *Pharmacoepidemiol Drug Saf* 2011;20:386-92. 許諾を得て転載)

2編 方法は Methods へ　結果は Results へ　解釈は Discussion へ

Before

Title

Plan 1) Efficacy of Low-dose Aspirin for Primary Prevention of Atherosclerotic Events Depends on Therapeutic Regimen of Diabetes: a post hoc analysis of the JPAD trial

Plan 2) Efficacy of Low-dose Aspirin for Primary Prevention of Atherosclerotic Events Depends on Severity of Diabetes: a post hoc analysis of the JPAD trial

Authors

Sadanori Okada[1], Takeshi Morimoto[2], Hisao Ogawa[3], Masafumi Nakayama[3], Shiro Uemura[1], Naofumi Doi[1], Akihide Jinnouch[4], Masako Waki[5], Hirofumi Soejima[3], Seigo Sugiyama[3], Mio Sakuma[2], Yasuhiro Akai[1], Masao Kanauchi[1], Yoshihiko Saito[1], for the Japanese Primary Prevention of Atherosclerosis With Aspirin for Diabetes (JPAD) Trial Investigators

Affiliations

[1]The First Department of Internal Medicine, Nara Medical University, 840 Shijo-cho, Kashihara, Nara, Japan 634-8522

[2]Center for Medical Education, Kyoto University Graduate School of Medicine, Konoe-cho, Yoshida, Sakyo-ku, Kyoto, Japan 606-8501

[3]Department of Cardiovascular Medicine, Graduate Medical School of Medical Science, Kumamoto University 1-1-1 Honjo, Kumamoto, Japan 860-8556

「効果」だとパッと読んだ際に単に「アスピリンの効果」の論文ととられてしまう．「異なる効果」というタイトルにすることで，読者は「ああ，効果の違いをみた論文なのだな」とすぐにわかる．

[4]Jinnouch Hospital, 6-2-3 Kyuhhonnji, Kumamoto, Japan 862-0976

[5]Division of Endocrinology and Metabolism, Department of Internal Medicine, Shizuoka City Hospital, 10-93, Ote-cho, Aoi-ku, Shizuoka, Japan 420-0630

Corresponding Author
Yoshihiko Saito, MD, PhD
The First Department of Internal Medicine, Nara Medical University
840 Shijo-cho, Kashihara, Nara, Japan 634-8522
Tel: xxxx, Fax: xxxx, Email: xxxx

Abstract

Aims/hypothesis
Recent meta-analyses report that low-dose aspirin is not effective on primary prevention of cardiovascular events in patients with diabetes. ＊ We tried to assess whether the efficacy of low-dose aspirin for primary prevention depends on therapeutic regimen of diabetes.

Methods
This study is a post hoc analysis of the JPAD trial: a multicenter, prospective, randomized, controlled, open-label, blinded-endpoint study in Japan. 2539 patients with type 2 diabetes and no previous cardiovascular disease were randomly assigned to the low-dose aspirin group (81 or 100mg daily) or the no aspirin group. A median follow-up was 4.37 years. We investigated the effect of low-dose aspirin on preventing atherosclerotic events in each diabetic treatment at baseline: insulin, n = 326; oral hypoglycemic agent (OHA), n = 1750; and diet alone, n = 463.

Results
The insulin group had the longest duration of diabetes, the highest level of HbA1C and fasting plasma glucose, and the highest prevalence of diabetic microangiopathies. In contrast, the diet alone group had the opposite characteristics. The incidence of atherosclerotic events was 26.6, 14.6, and 10.4 cases per 1000 person-years in the insulin, OHA, and diet alone groups, respectively. In the insulin and OHA groups, low-dose aspirin did not affect atherosclerotic events (insulin: HR, 1.19; 95%CI,

0.60-2.40; OHA: HR, 0.84; 95%CI, 0.57-1.24). In the diet alone group, low-dose aspirin significantly reduced atherosclerotic events in spite of the lowest event rates (HR: 0.21, 95%CI: 0.05-0.64).

Conclusions/interpretation
Low-dose aspirin reduced atherosclerotic events only in the diet alone group.

Trail registration
clinicaltrials.gov identifier, NCT00110448

Keywords
aspirin, type 2 diabetes, primary prevention, therapeutic regimen of diabetes

Abbreviations
ACCF	American College of Cardiology Foundation
AHA	American Heart Association
IQR	interquartile range
FPG	fasting plasma glucose
JDS	Japanese Diabetes Society
JPAD	Japanese Primary Prevention of Atherosclerosis with Aspirin for Diabetes
NGSP	National Glycoprotein Standardization Program
OHA	oral hypoglycemic agent
PHS	Physicians' Health Study
POPADAD	Prevention of Progression of Arterial Disease and Diabetes
PPP	Primary Prevention Project

Introduction

Cardiovascular disease is one of the major prognosis factors in patients with diabetes. Accumulated evidence has been shown that low-dose aspirin is effective in secondary prevention of cardiovascular events. Recently, the American Diabetic Association (ADA), the American Heart Association (AHA), and the American College of Cardiology Foundation (ACCF) jointly recommend the use of low-dose aspirin for primary prevention of cardiovascular events in patients with diabetes at high risk: aging (men over 50 years and women over 60 years) and one more

Introduction が長めであり，この部分は総説的なので削るべき．一方で直前のセンテンスは2次予防の話をしていて，この

additional risk factors, including smoking, hypertension, dyslipidemia, family history of cardiovascular disease, and alubuminuria. Previous studies suggest that low-dose aspirin is beneficial for primary prevention in general population at high risk; however its efficacy for patients with diabetes remains controversial.

Recently, two large clinical trials investigated whether low-dose aspirin reduced cardiovascular events in patients with diabetes and no cardiovascular disease. We have conducted the Japanese Primary Prevention of Atherosclerosis with Aspirin for Diabetes (JPAD) trial to examine efficacy of low-dose aspirin for primary prevention of atherosclerotic events in 2539 Japanese patients with type 2 diabetes. In the JPAD trial, we demonstrated that low-dose aspirin did not reduce atherosclerotic events. The overall event rate was 17 cases per 1000 person-years, which was one-third of the expected event rate at the start of the trial. Thus, there might be too few events to precisely estimate aspirin effect. The other trial: the Prevention of Progression of Arterial Disease and Diabetes (POPADAD) trial, which was registered 1276 patients with type 1 and type 2 diabetes in Scotland, also failed to document aspirin effect. The interpretation of the POPADAD trial was inconclusive because of the insufficient cardiovascular events and the low compliance of aspirin.

In general, patients with advanced stage of diabetes are considered as a high risk group. Previous epidemiological studies reported that pharmacological treatment of diabetes was associated with mortality. Notably, patients with insulin therapy increased mortality compared to that with oral hypoglycemic agent (OHA) therapy or diet alone. The ADA, AHA and ACCF recommend to use low-dose aspirin only for high risk diabetic patients. Therefore, the patients treated with insulin are expected to be most beneficial for low-dose aspirin therapy.

In this post-hoc analysis of the JPAD trial, we hypothesized that efficacy of low-dose aspirin depended on therapeutic regimen of diabetes. In this context, we investigated the effect of low-dose aspirin on preventing atherosclerotic events in each diabetic treatment at baseline: insulin (including combination with OHA therapy), OHA (excluding combination with insulin therapy), and diet alone (without usage of either insulin or OHA therapies).

Methods

Study design

The JPAD trial was a multicenter, prospective, randomized, open-label, blinded, end-point trial at 163 institutions throughout Japan. This trial was performed according to the Declaration of Helsinki and approved by the institutional review board at each participating hospital. Written informed consent was obtained from each participant.

The detail design of the JPAD trial was described previously. In brief, 2539 patients with type 2 diabetes and no history of cardiovascular disease (ages, between 30 and 85 years) were enrolled. The participants were randomly assigned to the aspirin group or the no aspirin group. 1262 patients in the aspirin group were assigned to take 81 mg or 100 mg of aspirin once daily. 1277 patients in the no aspirin group were also allowed to use antiplatelet therapy, including aspirin, if needed. All patients were allowed to use any concurrent treatment. ＊The median follow-up period was 4.37 years. A total of 193 patients were lost to follow-up, and data for those patients were censored at the day of last follow-up. The CONSORT diagram for the JPAD trial was presented previously.

＊ここにこの研究のメイン因子であるDMの管理（インスリン，OHA，食事）の定義を入れる．その結果である人数の分布は，Resultsの最初に入れる．
小数点以下は1桁で十分．

Definition of atherosclerotic events

The primary end point was any atherosclerotic event, which was a composite of sudden death; death from coronary, cerebrovascular, and aortic causes; nonfatal acute myocardial infarction; unstable angina; newly developed exertional angina; nonfatal ischemic and haemorrhagic stroke; transient ischemic attack; or nonfatal aortic and peripheral vascular disease during the follow-up period. All potential end points and haemorrhagic events were adjudicated by an independent committee on validation of data and events that was unaware of the group assignments.
＊

＊ResultsにあるHbA1cの計算方法はここに入れる．

Statistical analyses

Baseline characteristics were analyzed by ANOVA.
Efficacy comparisons were performed on the basis of time to the first event, according to the intention-to-treat principle, including all patients in the group to which they were randomized with patients lost to follow-up censored at the day of the last visit. Following the descriptive statistics, cumulative incidences of

efficacyの比較を記載する前に患者背景や記述統計を呈示するはずであり，それらの表現法や単純な比較の方法についての記載が必要．生存曲線を描くならその算出方法も記載を．

primary end points were estimated by the Kaplan-Meier method and differences between groups were assessed with the log-rank test. We used the Cox proportional hazards model to estimate HR of aspirin use along with 95%CI. ＊

All statistical analyses were conducted using ‥‥. P values of less than 0.05 were considered statistically significant.

Results

Baseline clinical characteristics

Table 1 shows the baseline clinical characteristics in each diabetic treatment. Overall mean age was 65 years, and the insulin group was a little younger (62 years) than the other groups (65 years). Median duration of diabetes was longest in the insulin group: 13.0 years in the insulin group, 7.2 years in the OHA group, and 3.5 years in the diet alone group. These data meant that the insulin group developed diabetes in the youngest age. It was reasonable for the highest prevalence of diabetic family history (relation within the third degree) in the insulin group. Glycemic control was worst in the insulin group and best in the diet alone group. Mean level of HbA1C was 8.1%, 7.6%, and 6.7% in the insulin, OHA, and diet alone groups, respectively. HbA1C level was presented by the calculated National Glycoprotein Standardization Program (NGSP) value, differently to Japanese Diabetes Society (JDS) value in the main analysis of the JPAD trial. NGSP value was converted from JDS value by the following formula: NGSP value (%) = JDS value (%) + 0.4%. The prevalence of diabetic microangiopathies (retinopathy, nephropathy, and neuropathy) was highest in the insulin group, and lowest in the diet alone group.

The complication of other cardiovascular risk factors was also shown in Table 1. The prevalence of hypertension and dyslipidemia was highest in the diet alone group. The use of statins was totally low: 18% in the insulin group, 27% in the OHA group, and 24% in the diet alone group. The habit of smoking and the family history of CVD were unchanged among the groups.

Incidence of atherosclerotic events in each diabetic treatment

The incidence of atherosclerotic events was 26.6, 14.6, and 10.4 cases per 1000 person-years in the insulin, OHA, and diet alone groups, respectively. The detail of atherosclerotic events was shown in Table 2. Both coronary artery disease and cerebrovascular disease were occurred most frequently in the insulin group. Peripheral vascular disease was low event rate and no difference among the three groups. Survival analysis showed that the rate of atherosclerotic events was significantly higher in the insulin group (log-rank test, P = 0.0013; Figure 1). These results demonstrated that the insulin group was actually at high cardiovascular risk.

	ここも具体的な数字を.

これも解釈なのでDiscussion へ.

Efficacy of low-dose aspirin in each diabetic treatment

Table 3 showed the baseline characteristics with or without aspirin therapy in each diabetic treatment. In the insulin group, low-dose aspirin did not affect the incidence of atherosclerotic events (HR, 1.19; 95%CI, 0.60-2.40; log-rank test, P = 0.61; Figure 2A). Similar results were observed in the OHA group (HR, 0.84; 95%CI, 0.57-1.24; log-rank test, P = 0.38; Figure 2B). On the other hand, in the diet alone group, low-dose aspirin significantly reduced atherosclerotic events in spite of the lowest event rates (HR: 0.21, 95%CI: 0.05-0.64; log-rank test, P = 0.0069; Figure 2C). *

＊多変量解析を入れるならこの場所.

Haemorrhagic events

In the JPAD trial, incidence of gastrointestinal bleeding and cerebral bleeding was very low (Table 4). They were similar between the aspirin and no aspirin group in each diabetic treatment.

Table 4 は情報量が少ないので text で十分.

Discussion

The major findings of this post hoc analysis are: 1) Japanese patients with type 2 diabetes treated with insulin had high incidence of atherosclerotic events; 2) low-dose aspirin reduced atherosclerotic events not in the insulin group but in the diet alone group. The insulin group had the longest duration of diabetes, the worst level of glycemic control, and the highest prevalence of diabetic microangiopathies at baseline. In contrast, the diet alone group had the opposite characteristics. There is no definitive criterion in severity of diabetes; however, it is usually classified according to the extent of vascular complications or the level of glycemic control. Thus, we could regard the insulin group as advanced stage of diabetes, and the diet alone group as early stage of diabetes. Our results might indicate that low-dose aspirin was most beneficial in early clinical stage of diabetes.

Previous clinical trials in general populations without precious cardiovascular disease showed that low-dose aspirin decreased the incidence of cardiovascular events; however, no trial provides definitive results in patients with diabetes. The Physicians' Health Study (PHS) was one of the major randomized, controlled trials to determine the effect of low-dose aspirin (325mg every other day) on primary prevention in 22071 healthy men. This study showed that low-dose aspirin reduced myocardial infarction by 44%, and it was terminated earlier than scheduled (a mean follow-up time: 5.0 years). In the subgroup analysis of the PHS, participants with diabetes had higher event rate of myocardial infarction than that without diabetes (diabetes, 37/533; no diabetes, 341/21513), but the efficacy of aspirin did not observed in patients with diabetes. The Primary Prevention Project (PPP) trial also assessed the difference in the low-dose aspirin (100mg daily) effect on primary prevention between people with and without diabetes. The PPP trial enrolled 4495 people who had at least one major cardiovascular risk factor, including 1031 people with diabetes. This trial was prematurely stopped by the ethical grounds and followed for a mean 3.6 years. In the main analysis of the PPP trial, low-dose aspirin lowered the incidence of cardiovascular events by 33%. In the diabetic group, low-dose aspirin did not reduce cardiovascular events in spite of higher event rate than that in nondiabetic group (event rate: diabetes, 44/1031; no diabetes, 81/3750). The subgroup analyses of both the PHS and the PPP trial were under-powered due to small number of diabetes and their premature stops; however, these results show that it is difficult to prove the benefit of low-dose aspirin therapy in patients with diabetes despite their high event rates.

Consistent with previous reports, we found that the insulin group had high atherosclerotic events and cardiovascular death in the JPAD trial. Despite their high event rates, we could not detect the benefit of low-dose aspirin in the insulin group. Our results may suggest the assumption that progression of diabetes attenuates the low-dose aspirin effect. In fact, platelet function has altered and activated in patients with diabetes.

A phenomenon that patients develop cardiovascular disease despite aspirin intake is often described as "aspirin resistance". It is considered as one of the mechanisms for insufficiency of low-

> Discussion が長いうえにこれらは全部「総説」となっている。このトピックを議論するより、本解析の主目的である治療法の差について十分に議論すべきである。また他の患者背景因子（例：腎機能）で、アスピリンの効果が違うことを紹介する。

dose aspirin. The detail of aspirin resistance remains obscure, but the underlying interindividual variability is consider to affect aspirin resistance. Several studies reported that the antiplatelet function by aspirin was lower in diabetic patients than in nondiabetic patients. The frequency of aspirin resistance was positively correlated with the level of HbA1C and fasting plasma glucose. The higher dose of aspirin improved aspirin resistance in patients with diabetes. In our study, poor glycemic control in the insulin group might diminish the aspirin effect via high-frequent aspirin resistance. Increasing dosage of aspirin may restore antipletlet function, but there are insufficient data of high-dose aspirin effect on prevention of cardiovascular events at this time.

The recent recommendation, stated by ADA, AHA and ACCF, is based on the concept whether the number of cardiovascular events prevented by low-dose aspirin (relative risk reduction of ~10%) is greater than the number of haemorrhagic events (1-5 per 1000 per year). Therefore, low-dose aspirin use depends on individual cardiovascular risk. The recommendation requires the accurate assessment of cardiovascular risk using a risk predictive tool for patients with diabetes, such as the UKPDS Risk Engine. It also describes that patients with higher cardiovascular risk should have greater absolute benefit of low-dose aspirin; however, there is imprecise evidence about this point. Additional evidence is required for the association between cardiovascular risk and aspirin effect.

Study strengths and limitations

Our project is the first report which estimates the effect of low-dose aspirin on primary prevention of cardiovascular events in therapeutic regimen of diabetes, as an indicator of diabetic severity. These results suggest clinical implications in the use of low-dose aspirin depending on clinical stage of diabetes. However, we have several limitations in this post-hoc analysis. ＊

Firstly, several OHAs are reported to prevent cardiovascular events (e.g. metformin, pioglitazone, and acarbose), but we analyzed the OHA group without discrimination of drug property. We could not assess the single-agent effect of such cardio-protective OHAs, because most of patients in the OHA group took sulfonylurea (81%) in the JPAD trial.

Secondly, the difference in the prevalence of hypertension among the diabetic treatments altered low-dose aspirin effect. Notably high prevalence in the diet alone group might enhance

＊主論文で述べた limitation は共通なので, ここに引用して省略する. そこから先の limitation はこの DM サブ解析特有なものに (例えば variable が時間で変化することなど).

aspirin effect. However, this relationship was uncertain, because the Thrombosis Prevention Trial, a randomized controlled trial to evaluate the benefit of low-dose aspirin therapy (75mg daily) for primary prevention of cardiovascular events, showed that low-dose aspirin was more effective for patients with lower blood pressure.

Finally, the small number of each diabetic treatment group, especially in the insulin group, was limited to conclude aspirin effect. As above mentioned, the JPAD trial had only one-third of the anticipated event rates. The subgroup amaysis of the JPAD trial is necessarily under-powered.

Conclusions

Recent meta-analyses, including data from the JPAD trial, report that low-dose aspirin is not effective on primary prevention of cardiovascular events in patients with diabetes. Our findings, however, indicate that low-dose aspirin reduced atherosclerotic events only in the diet alone group. These results might suggest that the efficacy of low-dose aspirin therapy is best in early stage of diabetes and diminishes along with progression of diabetes. Clinicians should make a decision based not only on conventional cardiovascular risk factors but also on clinical stage of diabetes to use low-dose aspirin for primary prevention. Further studies are needed to assess the benefit of low-dose aspirin therapy in each clinical stage of diabetes.

引用は，自分の結果からの conclusion ではない．

Acknowledgement（省略）

Disclosure（省略）

Appendix（省略）

Figure legends

Figure 1. Incidence of atherosclerotic events in each diabetic treatment group

Survival analysis showed that the rate of atherosclerotic events was significantly higher in the insulin group.

Figure 2. Efficacy of low-dose aspirin in each treatment group

In the insulin and OHA groups, low-dose aspirin did not affect the incidence of atherosclerocit events (A & B). On the other hand, in the diet alone group, low-dose aspirin significantly reduced atherosclerotic events in spite of the lowest event rates (C).

Table 1. Baseline Characteristics by treatments for diabetes

Treatment	Insulin	OHA	Diet alone	P value
n	326	1750	463	
Age, mean (SD), y	62 (10)	65 (10)	65 (10)	<0.0001
Male, n (%)	184 (56)	952 (54)	251 (54)	0.8
BMI, mean (SD), kg/m²	23 (4)	24 (4)	25 (4)	<0.0001
Duration of Diabetes, median (IQR), y	13.0 (7.7 - 19.1)	7.2 (3.3 - 12.1)	3.5 (1.0 - 7.6)	<0.0001
HbA1C, mean (SD), %	8.1 (1.5)	7.6 (1.3)	6.7 (0.8)	<0.0001
FPG, mean (SD), mol/L	8.77 (3.16)	8.27 (2.78)	7.22 (1.78)	<0.0001
Serum Creatinine, mean (SD), μ mol/L	71 (27)	71 (27)	71 (18)	0.8
Proteinuria, n (%)	58 (18)	243 (14)	48 (10)	0.01
Diabetic Retinopathy, n (%)	140 (43)	205 (12)	20 (4)	<0.0001
Diabetic Nephropathy, n (%)	66 (20)	220 (13)	36 (8)	<0.0001
Diabetic Neuropathy, n (%)	104 (32)	176 (10)	20 (4)	<0.0001
Diabetic Medications				
Sulfonylurea, n (%)	27 (8)	1420 (81)	0 (0)	<0.0001
α-Glycosidase Inhibitor, n (%)	88 (27)	748 (43)	0 (0)	<0.0001
Biguanide, n (%)	37 (11)	317 (18)	0 (0)	<0.0001
Thiazolidinedione, n (%)	9 (3)	119 (7)	0 (0)	<0.0001
Insulin, n (%)	326 (100)	0 (0)	0 (0)	—
Complications of Other Cardiovascular Risk Factors				
Hypertension, n (%)	156 (48)	983 (56)	334 (72)	<0.0001
Dyslipidemia, n (%)	132 (40)	953 (54)	260 (56)	<0.0001
History of Smoking, n (%)	146 (45)	731 (42)	182 (39)	0.3
Family History				
Diabetes, n (%)	153 (47)	731 (42)	155 (33)	0.0003
Coronary Artery Disease, n (%)	38 (12)	198 (11)	54 (12)	0.96
Stroke, n (%)	71 (22)	360 (21)	95 (21)	0.9

BMI was calculated as weight in kilograms divided by height in meters squared.
HbA1C level was presented by the calculated NGSP value, which was converted from the JDS value by the following formula: NGSP value (%) = JDS value (%) + 0.4%.
Hypertension is defined as a systolic BP ≥ 140 mmHg, a diastolic BP ≥ 90mmHg, or taking antihypertensive agents.
Dyslipidemia is defined as a total cholesterol level ≥ 5.7mmol/l, a fasting triglyceride level ≥ 1.7mmol/l, or taking antilipidemic agents.

Table 2. Atherosclerotic events in each diabetic treatment

Treatment	Insulin No. (%)	Insulin No. per 1000 Person-Years	OHA No. (%)	OHA No. per 1000 Person-Years	Diet Alone No. (%)	Diet Alone No. per 1000 Person-Years
Endpoint: all atherosclerotic events	33 (10)	26.6	102 (6)	14.6	19 (4)	10.4
Coronary Artery Disease	15 (5)	12.1	42 (2)	6.0	6 (1.3)	3.3
Fatal Coronary Artery Disease	4 (1.2)	3.2	1 (0.06)	0.1	0 (0)	0
Stroke	15 (5)	12.1	48 (3)	6.9	10 (2)	5.5
Fatal Stroke	0 (0)	0	5 (0.3)	0.7	1 (0.2)	0.5
Peripheral Artery Disease	3 (0.9)	2.4	12 (0.7)	1.7	3 (0.7)	1.6

セレクトして，textでもよい．

RCTなのでアスピリンの有無で差がないのは当たり前．アスピリンの有無をはずせばTable1と同じ．

Table 3. Baseline Characteristics by aspirin in each treatment

Treatment	Insulin Aspirin	Insulin No Aspirin	OHA Aspirin	OHA No Aspirin	Diet Alone Aspirin	Diet Alone No Aspirin
n	166	160	882	868	214	249
Age, mean (SD), y	63 (10)	61 (11)	65 (9)	64 (10)	65 (10)	65 (10)
Male, n (%)	96 (58)	88 (55)	478 (54)	474 (55)	132 (62)	119 (48)
BMI, mean (SD), kg/m²	24 (3)	23 (4)	25 (4)	24 (4)	25 (4)	24 ± 4
Duration of Diabetes, median (IQR), y	12.2 (7.7 - 19.4)	13.4 (7.5 - 18.6)	7.3 (3.3 - 12.1)	7.1 (3.4 - 12.3)	3.9 (1.0 - 8.5)	3.4 (1.1 - 6.5)
HbA1C, mean (SD), %	8.3 (1.7)	7.8 (1.2)	7.6 (1.4)	7.5 (1.2)	6.7 (0.8)	6.8 (0.8)
FPG, mean (SD), mmol/L	8.94 (3.27)	8.66 (3.05)	8.32 (2.83)	8.27 (2.78)	7.22 (1.72)	7.22 (1.78)
Serum Creatiine, mean (SD), μmol/L	71 (35)	71 (18)	71 (35)	71 (18)	71 (18)	71 (18)
Proteinuria, n(%)	28 (17)	30 (19)	131 (15)	112 (13)	19 (9)	29 (12)
Diabetic Retinopathy, n (%)	73 (44)	67 (42)	106 (12)	99 (11)	8 (4)	12 (5)
Diabetic Nephropathy, n (%)	31 (19)	35 (22)	120 (14)	100 (12)	18 (8)	18 (7)
Diabetic Neuropathy, n (%)	56 (34)	48 (30)	97 (11)	79 (9)	10 (5)	10 (4)

BMI was calculated as weight in kilograms divided by height in meters squared.
HbA1C level was presented by the calculated NGSP value, which was converted from the JDS value by the following formula: NGSP value (%) = JDS value (%) + 0.4%.

Table 4. Haemorrhagic events

Treatment	Insulin		OHA		Diet Alone	
	Aspirin	No Aspirin	Aspirin	No Aspirin	Aspirin	No Aspirin
Gastrointestinal Bleeding, *n* (%)	1 (0.6)	0 (0)	4 (0.5)	3 (0.4)	0 (0)	0 (0)
Haemorrhage Stroke, *n* (%)	1 (0.6)	1 (0.6)	5 (0.6)	4 (0.5)	0 (0)	2 (0.8)

textで十分.

References（省略）

Clinical Care/Education/Nutrition/Psychosocial Research
ORIGINAL ARTICLE

Differential Effect of Low-Dose Aspirin for Primary Prevention of Atherosclerotic Events in Diabetes Management

A subanalysis of the JPAD trial

SADANORI OKADA, MD[1]
TAKESHI MORIMOTO, MD, PHD[2]
HISAO OGAWA, MD, PHD[3]
MASAO KANAUCHI, MD, PHD[1]
MASAFUMI NAKAYAMA, MD, PHD[3]
SHIRO UEMURA, MD, PHD[1]
NAOFUMI DOI, MD, PHD[1]
HIDEAKI JINNOUCHI, MD, PHD[4]

MASAKO WAKI, MD, PHD[5]
HIROFUMI SOEJIMA, MD, PHD[3]
MIO SAKUMA, MD, PHD[2]
YOSHIHIKO SAITO, MD, PHD[1,6]
FOR THE JAPANESE PRIMARY PREVENTION OF ATHEROSCLEROSIS WITH ASPIRIN FOR DIABETES (JPAD) TRIAL INVESTIGATORS

OBJECTIVE—Recent reports showed that low-dose aspirin was ineffective in the primary prevention of cardiovascular events in diabetic patients overall. We hypothesized that low-dose aspirin would be beneficial in patients receiving insulin therapy, as a high-risk group.

RESEARCH DESIGN AND METHODS—This study is a subanalysis of the Japanese Primary Prevention of Atherosclerosis With Aspirin for Diabetes (JPAD) trial—a randomized, controlled, open-label trial. We randomly assigned 2,539 patients with type 2 diabetes and no previous cardiovascular disease to the low-dose aspirin group (81 or 100 mg daily) or to the no-aspirin group. The median follow-up period was 4.4 years. We investigated the effect of low-dose aspirin on preventing atherosclerotic events in groups receiving different diabetes management.

RESULTS—At baseline, 326 patients were treated with insulin, 1,750 with oral hypoglycemic agents (OHAs), and 463 with diet alone. The insulin group had the longest history of diabetes, the worst glycemic control, and the highest prevalence of diabetic microangiopathies. The diet-alone group had the opposite characteristics. The incidence of atherosclerotic events was 26.6, 14.6, and 10.4 cases per 1,000 person-years in the insulin, OHA, and diet-alone groups, respectively. In the insulin and OHA groups, low-dose aspirin did not affect atherosclerotic events (insulin: hazard ratio [HR] 1.19 [95% CI 0.60−2.40]; OHA: HR 0.84 [0.57−1.24]). In the diet-alone group, low-dose aspirin significantly reduced atherosclerotic events, despite the lowest event rates (HR 0.21 [0.05−0.64]).

CONCLUSIONS—Low-dose aspirin reduced atherosclerotic events predominantly in the diet-alone group and not in the insulin or OHA groups.

Diabetes Care 34:1277–1283, 2011

From the [1]First Department of Internal Medicine, Nara Medical University, Shijo-cho, Kashihara, Nara, Japan; the [2]Center for Medical Education, Kyoto University Graduate School of Medicine, Konoe-cho, Yoshida, Sakyo-ku, Kyoto, Japan; the [3]Department of Cardiovascular Medicine, Graduate School of Medical Science, Kumamoto University, Honjo, Kumamoto, Japan; the [4]Jinnouchi Hospital, Kuyhhonnji, Kumamoto, Japan; the [5]Department of Internal Medicine, Division of Endocrinology and Metabolism, Shizuoka City Hospital, Ote-cho, Aoi-ku, Shizuoka, Japan; and the [6]Department of Regulatory Medicine of Blood Pressure, Nara Medical University, Shijo-cho, Kashihara, Nara, Japan.
Corresponding author: Yoshihiko Saito, yssaito@naramed-u.ac.jp.
Received 29 December 2010 and accepted 21 March 2011.
DOI: 10.2337/dc10-2451. Clinical trial reg. no. NCT00110448, clinicaltrials.gov.
This article contains Supplementary Data online at http://care.diabetesjournals.org/lookup/suppl/doi:10.2337/dc10-2451/-/DC1.
© 2011 by the American Diabetes Association. Readers may use this article as long as the work is properly cited, the use is educational and not for profit, and the work is not altered. See http://creativecommons.org/licenses/by-nc-nd/3.0/ for details.

Cardiovascular disease is one of the major prognostic factors in patients with diabetes (1,2). Accumulated evidence has shown that low-dose aspirin is effective in the secondary prevention of cardiovascular events (3). Previous studies have suggested that low-dose aspirin is beneficial for primary prevention in members of the general population who are at high risk (4–8); however, its efficacy for patients with diabetes remains controversial (9).

Recently, two large clinical trials—the Japanese Primary Prevention of Atherosclerosis With Aspirin for Diabetes (JPAD) trial (10) and the Prevention of Progression of Arterial Disease and Diabetes (POPADAD) trial (11)—investigated whether low-dose aspirin reduced cardiovascular events in patients with diabetes but without cardiovascular disease. The JPAD trial, which was conducted by our research group, examined the efficacy of low-dose aspirin for primary prevention of atherosclerotic events in 2,539 Japanese patients with type 2 diabetes. The trial demonstrated that low-dose aspirin reduced atherosclerotic events by 20%, but statistical significance was not reached (10). The overall event rate was 17 cases per 1,000 person-years, which was one-third of the expected event rate at the start of the trial (10). Thus there might have been too few events to precisely estimate the effect of aspirin. The POPADAD trial, which registered 1,276 patients with either type 1 or type 2 diabetes in Scotland, also failed to document an effect of aspirin (11). It was determined that the POPADAD trial was inconclusive because of insufficient cardiovascular events and low compliance with aspirin therapy.

Recently, the American Diabetes Association (ADA), the American Heart Association (AHA), and the American College of Cardiology Foundation (ACCF) jointly recommended the use of low-dose aspirin for primary prevention of cardiovascular

Aspirin effect and diabetes management

events only in high-risk diabetic patients (12). Previous epidemiological studies have reported that diabetic patients undergoing insulin therapy have increased mortality compared with those receiving therapy with oral hypoglycemic agents (OHAs) or diet alone (13,14). Therefore, patients treated with insulin, defined to be a high-risk group, are considered to be the most likely to benefit from low-dose aspirin therapy.

In this subanalysis of the JPAD trial, we hypothesized that low-dose aspirin would be most beneficial for primary prevention in diabetic patients receiving insulin therapy. We investigated the effect of low-dose aspirin on preventing atherosclerotic events in groups categorized according to type of diabetes management at baseline.

RESEARCH DESIGN AND METHODS

Study design
The JPAD trial was a multicenter, prospective, randomized, open-label, blinded, end point trial conducted at 163 institutions throughout Japan. This trial was performed according to the Declaration of Helsinki and approved by the institutional review board at each participating hospital. Written informed consent was obtained from each participant before the trial.

The detailed design of the JPAD trial has been previously described (10). In brief, we enrolled 2,539 patients, aged between 30 and 85 years, with type 2 diabetes and no history of cardiovascular disease. The participants were randomly assigned to the aspirin group or the no-aspirin group. The 1,262 patients in the aspirin group were assigned to take 81 mg or 100 mg of aspirin once daily. The 1,277 patients in the no-aspirin group were allowed to use antiplatelet therapy, including aspirin, if needed. All patients were allowed to use any concurrent treatments.

In this subanalysis, we classified all participants into three subgroups according to the diabetes management at baseline: insulin, OHA, or diet alone. Patients with insulin and OHA combination therapy were included in the insulin group. The diet-alone group consisted of patients who used neither insulin nor OHAs. The median follow-up period was 4.4 years. A total of 193 patients were lost to follow-up, and data for those patients were censored at the day of last follow-up.

The Consolidated Standards of Reporting Trials (CONSORT) diagram for the JPAD trial was presented previously (10).

Definition of atherosclerotic events
The primary end point was the occurrence during the follow-up period of any atherosclerotic event, which was a composite of the following: death from coronary, cerebrovascular, and aortic causes; nonfatal acute myocardial infarction; unstable angina; newly developed exertional angina; nonfatal ischemic and hemorrhagic stroke; transient ischemic attack; and nonfatal aortic and peripheral vascular disease. All potential end points and hemorrhagic events (gastrointestinal bleeding and hemorrhagic stroke) were adjudicated by an independent committee that was blinded to the group assignments.

Presentation of hemoglobin A_{1c} level
Hemoglobin A_{1c} (HbA_{1c}) values were converted from the Japanese Diabetes Society (JDS) values used in the main analysis of the JPAD trial (10) into National Glycohemoglobin Standardization Program (NGSP) equivalent values. NGSP equivalent values were calculated using the following formula: NGSP equivalent value (%) = JDS value (%) + 0.4 (15).

Statistical analyses
Categorical variables were expressed as number and percentage and were compared with the χ^2 test. Continuous variables were expressed as mean values ± SDs unless otherwise indicated. Based on their distribution, continuous variables were compared using the Student *t* test or Wilcoxon rank sum test for two-group comparisons and ANOVA or Kruskal-Wallis test for three-group comparisons. Cumulative incidence was estimated by the Kaplan-Meier method, and differences were assessed with the log-rank test.

Efficacy comparisons were performed on the basis of time to the first event according to the intention-to-treat principle, with all patients included in the group to which they were randomized and with patients lost to follow-up censored at the day of the last visit. Cumulative incidences of end points were estimated by the Kaplan-Meier method, and differences between groups were assessed with the log-rank test. We used the Cox proportional hazard model to estimate the hazard ratio (HR) of aspirin use along with the 95% CI. We also developed multivariable Cox proportional hazard models to assess the effects of aspirin on atherosclerotic events adjusting for age (≥65 years), hypertension, dyslipidemia, and history of smoking to evaluate the robustness.

Statistical analyses were conducted by an independent statistician (T.M.) with the use of JMP 8.0 (SAS Institute, Cary, NC) software and SAS 9.2 (SAS Institute). P values of less than 0.05 were considered statistically significant.

RESULTS

Baseline clinical characteristics
At baseline, 326 patients were treated with insulin, 1,750 with OHAs, and 463 with diet alone (Table 1). The mean age was slightly lower in the insulin group (62 years) than the other groups (65 years). Mean BMI was lowest in the insulin group (23 kg/m^2) and highest in the diet-alone group (25 kg/m^2). Median duration of diabetes was longest in the insulin group: 13.0 years in the insulin group, 7.2 years in the OHA group, and 3.5 years in the diet-alone group. Mean levels of HbA_{1c} and fasting plasma glucose (FPG) were 8.1% and 8.77 mmol/L in the insulin group, 7.6% and 8.27 mmol/L in the OHA group, and 6.7% and 7.22 mmol/L in the diet-alone group. The prevalence of diabetic microangiopathies was highest in the insulin group (retinopathy, 43%; nephropathy, 20%; neuropathy, 32%) and lowest in the diet-alone group (retinopathy, 4%; nephropathy, 8%; neuropathy, 4%).

The frequency of other cardiovascular risk factors was also investigated at baseline (Table 1). The prevalence of hypertension and dyslipidemia was significantly higher in the diet-alone group (hypertension, 72%; dyslipidemia, 56%) than in the other two groups. The use of statins was low in all groups: 18, 27, and 24% in the insulin, OHA, and diet-alone groups, respectively. Smoking history and family history of cardiovascular diseases were similar among groups.

Atherosclerotic events in each diabetes management
The incidence of atherosclerotic events was 26.6, 14.6, and 10.4 cases per 1,000 person-years in the insulin, OHA, and diet-alone groups, respectively (Supplementary Table 1). Both coronary artery and cerebrovascular events occurred most frequently in the insulin group (coronary artery events, 12.1; cerebrovascular events, 12.1 cases per

Table 1—*Baseline characteristics by diabetes management*

Diabetes management	Insulin	OHA	Diet alone	P value
n	326	1,750	463	
Age (years)	62 (10)	65 (10)	65 (10)	<0.0001
Male, n (%)	184 (56)	952 (54)	251 (54)	0.8
BMI (kg/m^2)	23 (4)	24 (4)	25 (4)	<0.0001
Duration of diabetes (years)	13.0 (7.7–19.1)	7.2 (3.3–12.1)	3.5 (1.0–7.6)	<0.0001
HbA$_{1c}$ (%)	8.1 (1.5)	7.6 (1.3)	6.7 (0.8)	<0.0001
FPG (mmol/L)	8.77 (3.16)	8.27 (2.78)	7.22 (1.78)	<0.0001
Serum creatinine (μmol/L)	71 (27)	71 (27)	71 (18)	0.8
Proteinuria, n (%)	58 (18)	240 (14)	48 (10)	0.01
Diabetic retinopathy, n (%)	140 (43)	205 (12)	20 (4)	<0.0001
Diabetic nephropathy, n (%)	66 (20)	220 (13)	36 (8)	<0.0001
Diabetic neuropathy, n (%)	104 (32)	176 (10)	20 (4)	<0.0001
Diabetes medications, n (%)				
Sulfonylurea	27 (8)	1,420 (81)	0 (0)	<0.0001
α-Glycosidase inhibitor	88 (27)	748 (43)	0 (0)	<0.0001
Biguanide	37 (11)	317 (18)	0 (0)	<0.0001
Thiazolidinedione	9 (3)	119 (7)	0 (0)	<0.0001
Insulin	326 (100)	0 (0)	0 (0)	–
Family history of diabetes, n (%)	153 (47)	731 (42)	155 (33)	0.0003
Complications of other cardiovascular risk factors, n (%)				
Hypertension	156 (48)	983 (56)	334 (72)	<0.0001
Dyslipidemia	132 (40)	953 (54)	260 (56)	<0.0001
History of smoking	146 (45)	731 (42)	182 (39)	0.3
Family history of cardiovascular diseases, n (%)				
Coronary artery disease	38 (12)	198 (11)	54 (12)	0.96
Stroke	71 (22)	360 (21)	95 (21)	0.9

Data are mean (SD) or n (%); duration of diabetes data are median (interquartile range). BMI was calculated as weight in kilograms divided by height in meters squared. Hypertension was defined as systolic blood pressure ≥140 mmHg, diastolic blood pressure ≥90 mmHg, or therapy with antihypertensive agents. Dyslipidemia was defined as total cholesterol level ≥5.7 mmol/L, fasting triglyceride level ≥1.7 mmol/L, or therapy with antilipidemic agents.

1,000 person-years). There was a low incidence of peripheral vascular events among the three groups (insulin, 2.4; OHA, 1.7; diet alone, 1.6 cases per 1,000 person-years). Survival analysis showed that the rate of atherosclerotic events was significantly higher in the insulin group than those in the other groups (log-rank test, $P = 0.0013$; Fig. 1).

Efficacy of low-dose aspirin in each diabetes management

Participants were randomly assigned to the aspirin group or the no-aspirin group (Supplementary Table 2). In the insulin group, low-dose aspirin did not affect the incidence of atherosclerotic events (HR 1.19 [95% CI 0.60–2.40]; log-rank test, $P = 0.61$; Fig. 2A). Similar results were observed in the OHA group (HR 0.84 [0.57–1.24]; log-rank test, $P = 0.38$; Fig. 2B). On the other hand, in the diet-alone group, low-dose aspirin significantly reduced atherosclerotic events despite the fact that this group had the lowest atherosclerotic event rate (HR 0.21 [0.05–0.64]; log-rank test,

$P = 0.0069$; Fig. 2C). Adjusting for age, hypertension, dyslipidemia, and history of smoking, low-dose aspirin significantly reduced atherosclerotic events in the diet-alone group (HR 0.20 [0.06–0.68]; log-rank test, $P = 0.0099$) but not in the insulin or OHA groups (insulin: HR 1.0 [0.50–2.00], log-rank test, $P = 1.0$; OHA: HR 0.77 [0.52–1.14], log-rank test, $P = 0.20$).

Hemorrhagic events

The number of gastrointestinal bleeding and hemorrhagic strokes was very low overall and seemed similar between the aspirin and no-aspirin groups in each diabetes management. The number of gastrointestinal bleeding was one in the insulin group (this patient took aspirin) and seven in the OHA group (four in the aspirin group and three in the no-aspirin group). In the diet-alone group, no patients suffered from gastrointestinal bleeding. The number of hemorrhagic stroke was two in the insulin group (one in the aspirin group and one in the no-aspirin group), nine in the OHA group (five in the aspirin group and four in the

no-aspirin group), and two in the diet-alone group (all in the no-aspirin group).

CONCLUSIONS—The major findings of this subanalysis were as follows: Japanese patients with type 2 diabetes receiving insulin therapy had a high incidence of atherosclerotic events and low-dose aspirin reduced atherosclerotic events not in patients receiving insulin therapy but in patients treated with diet alone. These results were unchanged after adjusting for other cardiovascular risk factors.

The patients' baseline characteristics categorized by diabetes management obviously demonstrated the difference in diabetes status (Table 1). The insulin group was characterized by the youngest mean age (62 years) and the longest median duration of diabetes (13.0 years), which meant that patients in the insulin group developed diabetes at the youngest age among the three groups. In contrast, patients in the diet-alone group developed diabetes in recent years and at older age. The slightly but significantly low BMI in the insulin group (mean BMI, 23 kg/m^2)

Aspirin effect and diabetes management

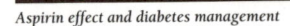

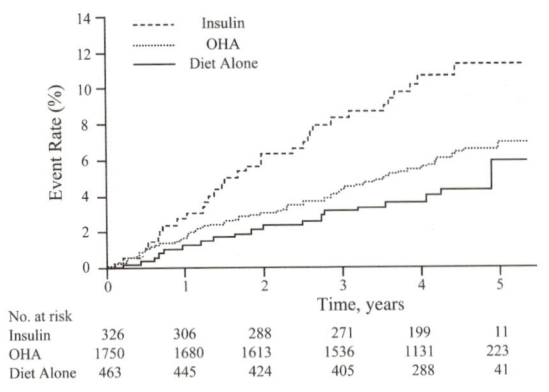

Figure 1—*Incidence of atherosclerotic events in each diabetes management. Survival analysis showed that the rate of atherosclerotic events was significantly higher in the insulin group (log-rank test, P = 0.0013).*

No. at risk	0	1	2	3	4	5
Insulin	326	306	288	271	199	11
OHA	1750	1680	1613	1536	1131	223
Diet Alone	463	445	424	405	288	41

might be a reflection of insufficient insulin secretion. The glycemic control was worst in the insulin group (mean levels of HbA_{1c} and FPG, 8.1% and 8.77 mmol/L) and best in the diet-alone group (mean levels of HbA_{1c} and FPG, 6.7% and 7.22 mmol/L). The prevalence of diabetic microangiopathies was highest in the insulin group (≥20%) and lowest in the diet alone group (<10%). There are no definitive criteria defining clinical stages of diabetes; however, it is usually classified according to the extent of vascular complications or the level of glycemic control. Thus we could regard the insulin group as demonstrating an advanced clinical stage of diabetes and the diet-alone group as demonstrating a less advanced or earlier clinical stage of diabetes than the insulin and OHA groups. Our results might indicate that low-dose aspirin was most beneficial in early clinical stages of diabetes, despite the lowest event rates.

Recently, we reported that a subanalysis of the JPAD trial showed a difference in low-dose aspirin effect on primary prevention of atherosclerotic events in renal function (16). In the study, reduced renal function in diabetic patients was significantly associated with high incidence of atherosclerotic events. Low-dose aspirin did not prevent atherosclerotic events in patients with an estimated glomerular filtration rate (eGFR) <60 mL/min/1.73 m² (HR 1.3 [95% CI 0.76–2.4]). On the other hand, in the patients with an eGFR of 60 to 89 mL/min/1.73 m², low-dose aspirin significantly reduced atherosclerotic events, despite low event rates (HR 0.57 [0.36–0.88]) (16). As in the current study, low-dose aspirin was not beneficial in patients with advanced stages of renal dysfunction and with high event rates but rather in those with early stages of renal dysfunction and with low event rates. These results suggest that progression of diabetes and diabetes complications (renal dysfunction) might attenuate the effect of low-dose aspirin.

The current recommendation of the ADA, AHA, and ACCF regarding the preventative use of aspirin in high-risk diabetic patients is based on the number of cardiovascular events prevented by low-dose aspirin (relative risk reduction of ~10%) being greater than the number of hemorrhagic events (1–5 cases per 1,000 person-years) (12). Therefore, low-dose aspirin use depends on individual cardiovascular risk. Because diabetic patients with higher cardiovascular risk should have greater absolute benefit from low-dose aspirin, our findings were unexpected and inconsistent with the recommendation. To confirm whether low-dose aspirin is really effective in high-risk or low-risk diabetic patients, further investigations are needed.

One possible mechanism of our findings is that events in patients with advanced clinical stages of diabetes are unpreventable because of overly advanced atherosclerotic lesions. Another possible mechanism is aspirin resistance in diabetic patients with poor glycemic control. Aspirin resistance is often described as a phenomenon whereby patients develop cardiovascular disease despite aspirin intake. The details surrounding aspirin resistance remain obscure, but it is thought to be affected by underlying interindividual variability (17). Increased platelet aggregation has been observed in patients with diabetes (18). Several studies have reported that aspirin's antiplatelet function is lower in diabetic patients than in nondiabetic patients (19) and that the frequency of aspirin resistance is positively correlated with the levels of HbA_{1c} and FPG (20). Higher aspirin doses have been shown to improve aspirin resistance in patients with diabetes (19). In our study, poor glycemic control in the insulin group might diminish the effects of aspirin via commonly occurring aspirin resistance. Increasing aspirin dosage may improve antiplatelet function, but there are insufficient data regarding the effect of high-dose aspirin on the prevention of cardiovascular events at this time (12). Combination therapy with aspirin and other antiplatelet agents, such as clopidogrel, suppresses platelet aggregation more strongly (19), but the benefit of dual antiplatelet therapy on primary prevention is also inconclusive (21).

The differing prevalence of other cardiovascular risk factors among patients in the various diabetic treatment groups might alter the low-dose aspirin effect on primary prevention of atherosclerotic events. In the diet-alone group, a high prevalence of hypertension (72%) and dyslipidemia (56%), high age (mean age, 65 years), mild overweight (mean BMI, 25 kg/m²), and mild glucose intolerance (mean levels of HbA_{1c} and FPG, 6.7% and 7.22 mmol/L) might indicate that these patients could be considered to have multiple cardiovascular risk factors rather than overt diabetes. In fact, previous clinical trials of primary prevention in patients with multiple cardiovascular risk factors showed that low-dose aspirin reduced cardiovascular events (5–7), whereas no trial provided a definitive conclusion regarding patients with diabetes (9–11). The Primary Prevention Project (PPP) trial reported a difference in the effect of low-dose aspirin on primary prevention between patients with and without overt diabetes (22). The PPP trial enrolled 4,495 patients with at least one major cardiovascular risk factor, including 1,031 patients with overt diabetes (FPG ≥7.8 mmol/L or treated with OHAs). This trial showed that low-dose aspirin lowered the incidence of cardiovascular events by 33% in total (7); however, in the diabetic group, low-dose aspirin did not reduce cardiovascular events despite 50% higher event rates (22). These reports might confirm that low-dose aspirin was beneficial in the diet-alone group, as a subset of patients in the early clinical stages of diabetes and with comorbid other cardiovascular risk factors.

Recent meta-analyses, including data from the JPAD trial, reported that low-dose aspirin is not effective in the primary prevention of cardiovascular events in patients with diabetes (9,23). Patients treated with insulin are at high risk for cardiovascular events; however, our findings indicated that low-dose aspirin reduced atherosclerotic events not in the insulin group but in the diet-alone group. These results suggest that low-dose aspirin therapy is most beneficial in early clinical stages of diabetes. When clinicians use low-dose aspirin in diabetic patients to prevent cardiovascular events, they should take into account not only conventional cardiovascular risk factors but also the clinical stage of diabetes. Further studies are needed to assess the effect of low-dose aspirin at each clinical stage of diabetes.

Study strengths and limitations
Our project is the first report to estimate the effect of low-dose aspirin on the primary prevention of atherosclerotic events in groups undergoing various diabetes management strategies. Our results suggest that the clinical impact of low-dose aspirin depends on the clinical stage of diabetes. However, this subanalysis has several limitations in addition to those reported in the main JPAD report (10).

First, we used the management of diabetes at baseline as a subgrouping variable. As with other variables, the management modality could change over time. Such changes could be especially frequent in the diet-alone and OHA groups as they begin to require more intensive treatment, and as a result the subgrouping might not be valid. Second, the small number of patients in each treatment group, especially in the insulin group, limited the certainty with which we could formulate conclusions regarding aspirin's effect. Larger studies are needed for definitive evaluation of the effect of aspirin in

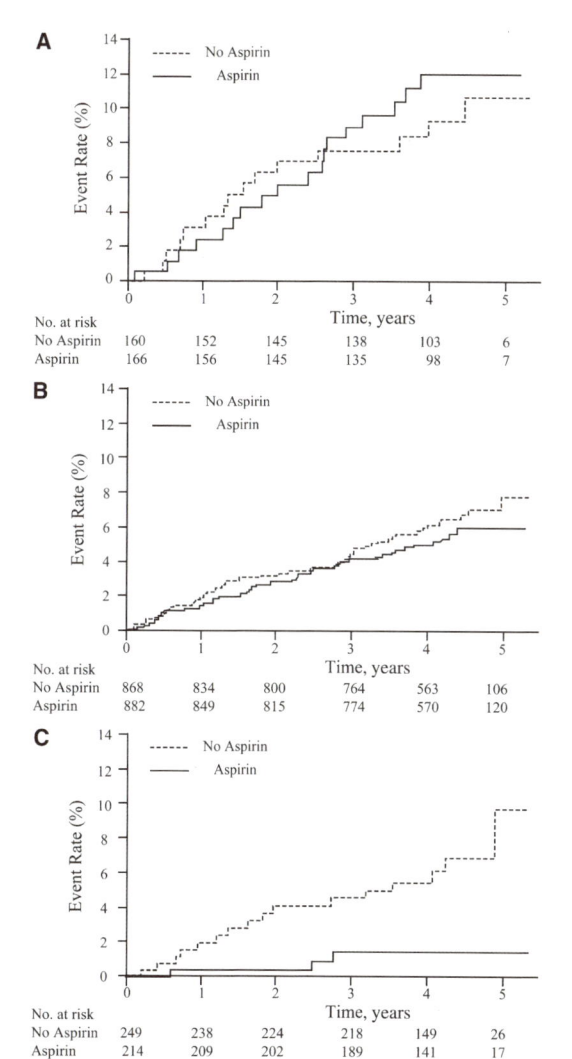

Figure 2—*Efficacy of low-dose aspirin on primary prevention of atherosclerotic events in each diabetes management. A and B: In the insulin (A) and OHA (B) groups, low-dose aspirin did not affect the incidence of atherosclerotic events (insulin: HR 1.19 [95% CI 0.60–2.40]; log-rank test, P = 0.61; OHA: HR 0.84 [0.57–1.24]; log-rank test, P = 0.38). C: In the diet-alone group, low-dose aspirin significantly reduced atherosclerotic events despite the lowest event rates (HR 0.21 [0.05–0.64]; log-rank test, P = 0.0069).*

patients treated with insulin. Third, several OHAs are reported to be beneficial for preventing cardiovascular events (e.g., metformin [24] and pioglitazone [25]), but we analyzed the OHA group without taking specific drug properties into account. Since most patients (81%) in the OHA group took sulfonylurea at baseline, we could not assess the single-agent effects of the cardioprotective OHAs. Finally, the number of hemorrhagic events was very low in both the aspirin and no-aspirin groups; however, the sample sizes were too small to estimate aspirin's side effects in the JPAD trial. Therefore, we could not make firm conclusions about the safety of low-dose aspirin based on our results.

Acknowledgments—This study was supported by the Ministry of Health, Labour and Welfare of Japan.

T.M. reported being on the Advisory Board of Pfizer, receiving research grants from Bayer and Eisai, and receiving lecturer's fees from Bayer, Eisai, Japan Tobacco, Kowa, Mitsubishi Tanabe, Otsuka, Pfizer, and Takeda for the past 2 years. H.O. reported receiving research grants from Abbott, Astellas, AstraZeneca, Banyu, Bayer, Boehringer Ingelheim, Chugai, Daiichi Sankyo, Dainippon Sumitomo, Eisai, Guidant Japan, Japan Lifeline, Kowa, Kyowa Hakko Kirin, Mitsubishi Tanabe, Mochida, Nihon Kohden, Novartis, Otsuka, Pfizer, sanofi-aventis, Schering-Plough, Sandoz, Sionogi, Takeda, Teijin, Toa Eiyo, Tyco Healthcare Japan, the Japan Heart Foundation, and the Smoking Research Foundation and receiving lecturer's fees from Astellas, Banyu, Bayer, Boehringer Ingelheim, Chugai, Daiichi Sankyo, Eisai, Kowa, Kyowa Hakko Kirin, Mitsubishi Tanabe, Novartis, Pfizer, sanofi-aventis, Schering-Plough, and Takeda for the past 2 years. M.S. reported receiving lecturer's fees from Otsuka and Pfizer for the past 2 years. Y.S. reported receiving research grant support from Astellas, AstraZeneca, Banyu, Baxter, Bayer Yakuhin, Daiichi Sankyo, Mitsubishi Tanabe, Novartis, Pfizer, and Takeda and receiving lecturer's fees from Banyu, Mitsubishi Tanabe, and Novartis for the past 2 years. No other potential conflicts of interest relevant to this article were reported.

S.O. conducted the trial, researched data, contributed to discussion, and wrote, reviewed, and edited the manuscript. T.M. researched and managed data, contributed to discussion, and wrote, reviewed, and edited the manuscript. H.O. contributed to discussion and reviewed and edited the manuscript. M.K. conducted the trial and researched data. M.N. researched data. S.U. contributed to discussion. N.D., H.J., and M.W. researched data. H.S. researched data and contributed to discussion. M.S. researched data, contributed to discussion, and wrote, reviewed, and edited the manuscript. Y.S. conducted the trial, researched data, contributed to discussion, and wrote, reviewed, and edited the manuscript.

Parts of this study were presented at the 2010 Scientific Sessions of the AHA, Chicago, Illinois, 13–17 November 2010.

The authors thank H. Ueshima (Shiga University of Medical Science, Otsu, Japan), H. Imura (Foundation for Biomedical Research and Innovation, Kobe, Japan), and K. Kimura (Yokohama City University Medical Center, Yokohama, Japan) for their attending the Safety Monitoring Board in the JPAD trial; I. Masuda (Higashiyama-Takeda Hospital, Kyoto, Japan) for his validation of data and events; and M. Ohtorii (Kyoto University, Kyoto, Japan), E. Miyake (Kyoto University, Kyoto, Japan), A. Mizutani (Kyoto University, Kyoto, Japan), and K. Sakamoto (Kyoto University, Kyoto, Japan) for their managing of data. The authors also thank Y. Akai (Nara Medical University, Kashihara, Japan) and Y. Yoshimasa (Yoshimasa-Naika Clinic, Toyonaka, Japan) for discussion and M. Nagahiro (Kumamoto University, Kumamoto, Japan), Y. Wada (Nara Medical University, Kashihara, Japan), T. Higashi (Nara Medical University, Kashihara, Japan), Y. Kouno (Nara Medical University, Kashihara, Japan) and M. Miyagwa (Nara Medical University, Kashihara, Japan) for their secretarial work.

References

1. Brun E, Nelson RG, Bennett PH, et al.; Verona Diabetes Study. Diabetes duration and cause-specific mortality in the Verona Diabetes Study. Diabetes Care 2000;23: 1119–1123
2. Roper NA, Bilous RW, Kelly WF, Unwin NC, Connolly VM; South Tees Diabetes Mortality Study. Cause-specific mortality in a population with diabetes: South Tees Diabetes Mortality Study. Diabetes Care 2002;25:43–48
3. Baigent C, Blackwell L, Collins R, et al.; Antithrombotic Trialists' (ATT) Collaboration. Aspirin in the primary and secondary prevention of vascular disease: collaborative meta-analysis of individual participant data from randomised trials. Lancet 2009;373:1849–1860
4. Final report on the aspirin component of the ongoing Physicians' Health Study. Steering Committee of the Physicians' Health Study Research Group. N Engl J Med 1989;321:129–135
5. Hansson L, Zanchetti A, Carruthers SG, et al.; HOT Study Group. Effects of intensive blood-pressure lowering and low-dose aspirin in patients with hypertension: principal results of the Hypertension Optimal Treatment (HOT) randomised trial. Lancet 1998;351:1755–1762
6. Thrombosis prevention trial: randomised trial of low-intensity oral anticoagulation with warfarin and low-dose aspirin in the primary prevention of ischaemic heart disease in men at increased risk, The Medical Research Council's General Practice Research Framework. Lancet 1998; 351:233–241
7. de Gaetano G; Collaborative Group of the Primary Prevention Project. Low-dose aspirin and vitamin E in people at cardiovascular risk: a randomised trial in general practice. Lancet 2001;357:89–95
8. Ridker PM, Cook NR, Lee IM, et al. A randomized trial of low-dose aspirin in the primary prevention of cardiovascular disease in women. N Engl J Med 2005; 352:1293–1304
9. De Berardis G, Sacco M, Strippoli GF, et al. Aspirin for primary prevention of cardiovascular events in people with diabetes: meta-analysis of randomised controlled trials. BMJ 2009;339:b4531
10. Ogawa H, Nakayama M, Morimoto T, et al.; Japanese Primary Prevention of Atherosclerosis With Aspirin for Diabetes (JPAD) Trial Investigators. Low-dose aspirin for primary prevention of atherosclerotic events in patients with type 2 diabetes: a randomized controlled trial. JAMA 2008;300:2134–2141
11. Belch J, MacCuish A, Campbell I, et al.; Prevention of Progression of Arterial Disease and Diabetes Study Group; Diabetes Registry Group; Royal College of Physicians Edinburgh. The Prevention Of Progression of Arterial Disease And Diabetes (POPADAD) trial: factorial randomised placebo controlled trial of aspirin and antioxidants in patients with diabetes and asymptomatic peripheral arterial disease. BMJ 2008;337:a1840
12. Pignone M, Alberts MJ, Colwell JA, et al.; American Diabetes Association; American Heart Association; American College of Cardiology Foundation. Aspirin for primary prevention of cardiovascular events in people with diabetes: a position statement of the American Diabetes Association, a scientific statement of the American Heart Association, and an expert consensus document of the American College of Cardiology Foundation. Diabetes Care 2010;33: 1395–1402
13. Muggeo M, Verlato G, Bonora E, et al. The Verona diabetes study: a population-based survey on known diabetes mellitus prevalence and 5-year all-cause mortality. Diabetologia 1995;38:318–325
14. Stengård JH, Tuomilehto J, Pekkanen J, et al. Diabetes mellitus, impaired glucose tolerance and mortality among elderly men: the Finnish cohorts of the Seven Countries Study. Diabetologia 1992;35: 760–765
15. The Committee of Japan Diabetes Society on the diagnostic criteria of diabetes mellitus. Report of the Committee on the classification and diagnostic criteria of diabetes mellitus. J Jpn Diabetes Soc 2010;53: 450–467

16. Saito Y, Morimoto T, Ogawa H, et al.; Japanese Primary Prevention of Atherosclerosis With Aspirin for Diabetes Trial Investigators. Low-dose aspirin therapy in patients with type 2 diabetes mellitus and reduced glomerular filtration rate: subanalysis from the JPAD trial. Diabetes Care 2011;34:280–285
17. Mansour K, Taher AT, Musallam KM, Alam S. Aspirin resistance. Adv Hematol 2009;2009:937352
18. Colwell JA, Halushka PV, Sarji K, Levine J, Sagel J, Nair RM. Altered platelet function in diabetes mellitus. Diabetes 1976;25 (Suppl. 2):826–831
19. DiChiara J, Bliden KP, Tantry US, et al. The effect of aspirin dosing on platelet function in diabetic and nondiabetic patients: an analysis from the aspirin-induced platelet effect (ASPECT) study. Diabetes 2007;56:3014–3019
20. Ertugrul DT, Tutal E, Yildiz M, et al. Aspirin resistance is associated with glycemic control, the dose of aspirin, and obesity in type 2 diabetes mellitus. J Clin Endocrinol Metab 2010;95:2897–2901
21. Wang TH, Bhatt DL, Fox KA, et al.; CHARISMA Investigators. An analysis of mortality rates with dual-antiplatelet therapy in the primary prevention population of the CHARISMA trial. Eur Heart J 2007;28:2200–2207
22. Sacco M, Pellegrini F, Roncaglioni MC, Avanzini F, Tognoni G, Nicolucci A; PPP Collaborative Group. Primary prevention of cardiovascular events with low-dose aspirin and vitamin E in type 2 diabetic patients: results of the Primary Prevention Project (PPP) trial. Diabetes Care 2003;26:3264–3272
23. Pignone M, Williams CD. Aspirin for primary prevention of cardiovascular disease in diabetes mellitus. Nat Rev Endocrinol 2010;6:619–628
24. UK Prospective Diabetes Study (UKPDS) Group. Effect of intensive blood-glucose control with metformin on complications in overweight patients with type 2 diabetes (UKPDS 34). Lancet 1998;352:854–865
25. Dormandy JA, Charbonnel B, Eckland DJ, et al.; PROactive investigators. Secondary prevention of macrovascular events in patients with type 2 diabetes in the PROactive Study (PROspective pioglitAzone Clinical Trial In macroVascular Events): a randomised controlled trial. Lancet 2005;366:1279–1289

(Okada S, et al.：Differential effect of low-dose aspirin for primary prevention of atherosclerotic events in diabetes management: a subanalysis of the JPAD trial. Japanese Primary Prevention of Atherosclerosis With Aspirin for Diabetes Trial Investigators. *Diabetes Care* 2011;34:1277-83. 許諾を得て転載）

3編 受動態より能動態を使う ％は分子分母も併記する

Before

Title
Association of symptom-onset-to-balloon time with long-term outcome in patients with ST-segment elevation myocardial infarction undergoing primary percutaneous coronary intervention

> このままではわかりにくい．onset-to-balloon や，国際的な door-to-balloon を考慮する．

Names of Authors
Hiroki Shiomi, M.D.[1], ……

Institutions
[1] Department of Cardiovascular Medicine, Graduate School of Medicine, Kyoto University, Kyoto, Japan

Names of grants
This study was supported by the Pharmaceuticals and Medical Devices Agency (PMDA) in Japan.

Address for correspondence
Takeshi Kimura
Department of Cardiovascular Medicine, Graduate School of Medicine, Kyoto University
54 Shogoin Kawahara-cho, Sakkyo-ku, Kyoto 606-8507 Japan
TEL: xxxx FAX: xxxx
E-mail : xxxx

Total word count
2997, 5 tables, 5 figures

Abstract

Context

The impact of symptom-onset-to-balloon (O2B) time on long-term outcome in patients with ST-segment elevation myocardial infarction (STEMI) undergoing primary percutaneous coronary intervention (PCI) has not been adequately established.

Objective

To evaluate the relationship of O2B time with long-term outcome in patients with STEMI undergoing primary PCI.

Design, setting, and patients

An observational study on 3455 STEMI patients with primary PCI within 24 hours of symptom onset in a large scale cohort of acute myocardial infarction in Japan.

Main outcome measures

A composite of death and congestive heart failure (CHF) admission, compared by O2B time and door-to-balloon (D2B) time.

Results

Compared with an O2B time greater than 3 hours, an O2B time of less than 3 hours was associated with better clinical outcomes in terms of mortality (10.7% vs 14.7% at 3 years; p =0.01) and a composite of death and CHF admission (13.8% vs 19.3% at 3 years; p =0.0007). A D2B time of less than 90 minutes was associated with a lower incidence of a composite of death and CHF admission in patients presenting within 2 hours of symptom onset (12.0% vs17.7% at 3 years; p =0.02), but not in those presenting later (19.7% vs18.7% at 3 years; p =0.4). Multivariate Cox proportional analysis revealed the relationship of a short O2B (≤ 3 hours) with a better outcome in terms of a composite of all-cause death and CHF admission (adjusted hazard ratio (HR) 0.73; 95% confidence interval (C.I) 0.59 - 0.92; p = 0.007).

Conclusions

A symptom-onset-to-balloon (O2B) time of less than 3 hours was associated with better clinical outcomes in terms of a composite of death and CHF admission, and the impact of a door-to-balloon (D2B) time of less than 90 minutes on better outcomes was observed only in patients presenting within 2 hours of symptom onset.

Introduction

In recent decades, in-hospital mortality after acute myocardial infarction has dramatically decreased to less than 10% because of establishment of coronary care units (CCUs), improvements in medical therapy, and widespread use of early reperfusion therapy. Above all, primary percutaneous coronary intervention (PCI) is considered to play a central role in treatment of ST segment elevation myocardial infarction (STEMI). The current ACC/AHA guideline recommends door-to-balloon (D2B) time of less than 90 minutes as Class 1 recommendation. Even today, however, some controversies remain regarding time to treatment and outcomes in patients with STEMI undergoing primary PCI. A correlation between symptom-onset-to-balloon (O2B) time and mortality was originally observed in several previous registries but not in NRMI (National Registry of Myocardial Infarction) which consists of more than 20,000 patients in United States. In addition, many large-scale registries that consisted of several thousand patients reported that the benefit of a D2B time of less than 90 minutes was observed only in patients with early presentation (2 or 3 hours after symptom onset), and not in patients with delayed presentation. Still other registries have reported that the effect of a D2B time of less than 90 minutes was not affected by the time from symptom onset to presentation8,9. Finally, NRMI registries have reported that the benefit of early reperfusion is not influenced by patients' risk profiles, although other registries have reported that the benefit is limited to only high-risk patients and did not extend to low-risk patients.

The purpose of this study was to help resolve these conflicting issues in a large-scale cohort of acute myocardial infarction (AMI) in Japan.

この文は総論的で，今回の主たる対象であるSTEMIやPCIを強調しづらい．次のセンテンスを前にもってくるべき．

Methods

Study design and Patient Population

The Coronary REvascularization Demonstrating Outcome Study in Kyoto (CREDO-Kyoto) AMI registry is a physician-initiated non-company sponsored multi-center registry that enrolled consecutive AMI patients undergoing coronary revascularization within 7 days of symptom onset across 26 community and tertiary hospitals in Japan between January 2005 and December 2007.

Of the 5429 patients in the CREDO-Kyoto AMI registry, 195 patients underwent coronary artery bypass graft surgery and were excluded from the current analysis. In the remaining 5234 patients, 4444 patients had an admission diagnosis of STEMI. The current study population consisted of the 3455 patients with STEMI who underwent PCI within 24 hours for whom the O2B time were available (Figure 1).

Definitions of Clinical Characteristics and Endpoints

Baseline clinical characteristics such as prior myocardial infarction (MI), heart failure (HF), hypertension, current smoking, atrial fibrillation, chronic obstructive pulmonary disease (COPD), liver cirrhosis and malignancy were regarded as present when these diagnoses were recorded in the hospital charts. Elderly patients were defined as those patients ≥ 75 years of age. Diabetes was defined as treatment with oral hypoglycemic agents and/or insulin, a prior clinical diagnosis of diabetes, a glycated hemoglobin level ≥ 6.5%, or blood glucose level ≥ 200 mg/dl (although blood glucose test results in the acute phase of AMI were not used for the diagnosis of diabetes). Prior stroke was defined as infarction or intracranial bleeding with neurological symptoms lasting > 24 hours. Peripheral vascular disease was regarded to be present when carotid, aortic, or other peripheral vascular diseases were being treated or scheduled for surgical or endovascular interventions. Left ventricular ejection fraction (LVEF) was measured either by contrast left ventriculography or echocardiography, and low LVEF was defined as LVEF ≤ 40%. Renal function was expressed as estimated glomerular filtration rate (e-GFR) calculated by the Modification of Diet in Renal Disease formula modified for Japanese patients. Renal insufficiency defined as present in patients on dialysis and/or those with an e-GFR ≤ 30 mL*min-1*1.73mm-2. Anemia was defined as blood hemoglobin level less than 11.0g/dl. Thrombocytopenia was defined as a platelet count <100*109/L.

During the follow-up, death was regarded as cardiac in origin unless obvious non-cardiac causes could be identified. MI was defined according to the definition in the Arterial Revascularization Therapy Study. Scheduled staged PCI procedures during the index hospitalization or performed within 3 months of the initial procedure were not regarded as follow-up events but were included in the index procedure. Events such as cardiac death and MI were adjudicated by a clinical event committee. CHF admission was defined as hospitalization due to worsening CHF requiring intravenous drug therapy.

Outcome measures of the current analysis were long-term mortality and a composite endpoint of all-cause death and CHF admission (death/CHF), and the principal variables were O2B time and D2B time.

Data Collection and Follow-up

Demographic, angiographic, and procedural data were collected from hospital charts or hospital databases according to pre-specified definitions by independent experienced clinical research coordinators from the study management center. Follow-up data were obtained over 3 years, from hospital charts or by contacting patients or referring physicians. Because final data collection for follow-up events was initiated on July 1st, 2009, follow-up events were censored on this date. The median follow-up duration was 922 days (with an inter-quartile range [IQR]: 633-1226 days). Complete 1-year follow-up information was obtained in 3303 patients (95.6%) of 3455 study patients.

The relevant review boards or ethics committees in all 26 participating centers approved the study protocol. Obtaining written informed consent from the patients were waived because of the retrospective nature of the study; however, we excluded those patients who refused participate in the study when contacted at follow-up. This strategy is in agreement with the guidelines for epidemiological studies issued by the Ministry of Health, Labor and Welfare of Japan.

Statistical Analysis

Continuous variables are presented as the mean ± SD or median with IQR, and categorical variables are expressed as numbers and percentages. Categorical variables were compared with the Chi-square test when appropriate; otherwise, a Fisher exact test was used. Continuous variables were compared with Student's t-test or Wilcoxon rank-sum test based on the distribution. Cumulative incidences of clinical event rates were estimated by the Kaplan-Meier method, and differences were assessed with the log-rank test.

We divided the patients into two groups according to their O2B time to assess the effect of a short O2B time on clinical outcome. The cutoff point of O2B time was set at 3 hours in light of previously reported date and the distribution of O2B times in this cohort (eFigure 1). We also divided the patients into two groups according to time to presentation after symptom onset. The cutoff point of this time was set at 90 minutes, following the recommendation in the current ACC/AHA guideline.

As a subgroup analysis, we compared the effects of an O2B time less than 3 hours among the different risk profiles of the patients, such as CHF, age, anterior MI, renal insufficiency, and multi-vessel disease (MVD).

We used a multivariable Cox proportional-hazards model stratified by centers to estimate the hazard ratio (HR) of O2B time for a composite of death/CHF by adjusting for 39 clinically relevant variables (listed in Table 1). Multivariate analysis for D2B time stratified by the time to presentation (≤ 2 hours after symptom onset or later) was also performed in the same manner. The cutoff point was set at 2 hours in light of previously reported date and the distribution of O2B times in this cohort (eFigure 2). The same Cox proportional hazard models were developed for D2B in the patients with early presentation (≤ 2 hours after symptom onset) and in those with delayed presentation (> 2 hours after symptom onset) with the same independent variables other than O2B time. We added an interaction variable between the time to presentation (≤ 2 / > 2 hours after symptom onset) and D2B time (≤ 90 / > 90 minutes) in the model of the entire study population to assess whether the effect size of D2B time ≤ 90 minutes relative to D2B time > 90 minutes was different between the patients with early presentation and those with delayed presentation.

All analyses were conducted by a physician (H.S.) and a statistician (T.M.) using JMP 7 and SAS 9.2 (SAS Institute Inc., Cary, NC), and reported p values were two-sided. A p value < 0.05 was regarded as statistically significant.

Results

Baseline Characteristics
*

Baseline characteristics of the patients are shown in Table 1. Elderly patients, prior stroke, and anemia were more common in the delayed O2B group (O2B time > 3 hours), whereas the short O2B group (O2B time ≤ 3 hours) included more patients with low body mass index (BMI), who were current smokers and had unstable hemodynamics such as cardiac arrest, cardiogenic shock at presentation. Mechanical supports such as intra-aortic balloon pumping (IABP) and Percutaneous cardio-pulmonary support (PCPS) were more common in the delayed O2B group.

Regarding time to treatment, the median onset to presentation time in the short O2B group was 1.0 hours (IQR: 0.7-1.4 hours) and that in the delayed O2B group was 3.7 hours (IQR: 2.3-7.5 hours). The median O2B time in the short O2B group and the delayed O2B group were 2.3 hours (1.9-2.7 hours) and 5.5 hours (IQR: 4.0-9.4 hours), respectively. The rate of achievement of a D2B time of less than 90 minutes was 66 % in the short O2B group and 45 % in the delayed O2B group (p <0.0001).

> onset-to-balloon と書けば当たり前なので不要.
> 主たる結果なので前へ．また short と delayed に分ける前の全体のデータが必要.

In terms of lesion characteristics, the delayed O2B group included more patients with MVD, lateral infarction, posterior infarction, and a culprit lesion of the left circumflex (LCx), although a culprit lesion of Left main coronary artery (LMCA) and use of thrombectomy was higher in the short O2B group (Table 2).

Regarding medication at hospital discharge, the majority of patients in both groups received dual antiplatelet therapy (Table 3). The use of statins and beta blockers was significantly more prevalent in the short O2B group, whereas cilostazol was more often used in the delayed O2B group.

Relationship of time to treatment and clinical outcomes

The group with an O2B time of ≤ 3 hours group had a lower long-term mortality compared with the other groups (Figure 2A, 2C). A short O2B time was clearly beneficial in terms of a composite of death/CHF according to each time period (Figure 2D).

> Figure だけでなく，event 数や母集団の分子分母もほしい.

Regarding D2B time, there was no significant difference in mortality or in a composite of death/CHF in the entire cohort (Figure3A, 3B). When stratified by time to presentation, however, a D2B time of less than 90 minutes had a significant impact on patients presenting early, but did not have a significant impact on patients presenting later (Figure3C, 3D).

Subgroup analysis according to risk profile of the patients

In patients presenting with CHF, a short O2B time (O2B time

≤ 3 hours) was associated with a better clinical outcome (unadjusted HR: 0.71, 95%C.I: 0.56-0.89, p = 0.003), although the benefit of a short O2B time was also observed in patients without CHF (Unadjusted HR: 0.64, 95%C.I: 0.45-0.90, p = 0.01; Figure 4A, 4B). Regarding patient age, a tendency towards a better clinical outcome was observed in both elderly and relatively younger patients (Figure 4C, 4D). In all subgroups, the absolute risk reduction of a short O2B time was greater in high-risk patients, although the relative risk reduction was almost similar (Figure 4, 5).

Multivariate analysis for time to treatment

As shown in Table 4, an O2B time of ≤ 3 hours was an independent predictor for a composite of death/CHF (adjusted HR: 0.73, 95%C.I: 0.59-0.92, p = 0.007). There were interactions between D2B time (>/≤ 90 minutes) and the time to presentation (≤/> 2 hours after symptom onset)(interaction p = 0.02). A D2B time ≤ 90 minutes was an independent predictor for lower incidence of a composite of death/CHF only in patients with early presentation (adjusted HR: 0.54, 95% C.I: 0.35-0.85, p = 0.008), but not in those with delayed presentation (adjusted HR: 1.57, 95% C.I: 1.12-2.18, p = 0.008). ※Regarding the other clinically relevant factors, culprit DES use, thrombectomy and use of medication recommended by the guideline were associated with a better clinical outcome after adjusting for confounding factors, whereas many severe comorbidities and lesion characteristics, such as CHF, prior myocardial infarction, dialysis, malignancy, and target of unprotected LMCA, were associated with a poor clinical outcome (Table 4, 5).

> このinteractionは後ろのモデルのinteractionであり，＊に記載する．

Comment

The main findings of the current analysis are as follows: (1) a symptom-onset-to-balloon (O2B) time of less than 3 hours was associated with lower long-term mortality in patients with STEMI undergoing primary PCI; (2) The benefit of a D2B time of less than 90 minutes on clinical outcome was limited to patients with early presentation; (3) the absolute risk reduction of a short O2B time was greater in high-risk patients, although similar benefits were observed in low-risk patients.

> このlong-termが3年の研究から得られた知見であることを明記する．

The current analysis demonstrated a clear relationship between a short O2B time, especially O2B time of less than 3 hours, and lower long-term mortality in patients with STEMI undergoing primary PCI. This result is consistent with the previously reported pathophysiological observation that the effect of reperfusion on myocardial salvage is markedly decreased within 2 or 3 hours after onset of infarction. The NRMI registry reported no correlation between O2B time and mortality, although D2B time was associated with lower mortality. They suggested that they could not observe the correlation between O2B time and mortality because of patients' recall bias for symptom onset, survivor bias and variety in the time course of developing myocardial necrosis. We cannot completely exclude the idea that these factors might influence the correlation between O2B time and mortality. However, their result itself suggested that correlation between D2B time and a better outcome was due not to the effect of early reperfusion, but rather to the situation that resulted in a short D2B time, such as high quality of general treatment in the hospitals with a short D2B time or patient characteristics that allowed early reperfusion. The D2B time is part of the O2B time, which represents the total ischemic time, and we cannot theoretically exclude the influence of onset time on mortality regardless of the time index used. We speculate that we observed a clear correlation between the O2B time and a better clinical outcome for several reasons: the majority of the patients in this cohort presented early; unclear onset time was treated as a missing value because research coordinators collected personal date from hospital charts; and most importantly, the endpoint was long-term outcome instead of in-hospital mortality. Indeed, in-hospital mortality was not significantly different between the short O2B group and the delayed O2B group, although in-hospital mortality for those with a D2B time of less than 90 minutes tended to be lower than for those with D2B time of more than 90 minutes in patients with early presentation. An accurate indicator of the progress of developing ischemia would be an ideal tool, but it does not yet exist in daily clinical practice. Therefore, the current guideline has emphasized the target of a D2B time of less than 90 minutes, and the rate at which this is achieved has improved in recent years. By contrast, Flynn et al. reported that efforts to reduce the D2B time had not reduced mortality rates. This finding may reflect that the D2B time represents only part of the total ischemic time. Therefore, it is important to evaluate patients and select treatments on the basis of total ischemic time, and the result of current analysis offers meaningful information, although patients with unclear symptom onset times will exist in daily clinical practice.

Furthermore, this study was able to separate the benefit of early reperfusion according to each O2B time period, by evaluating a composite of death and CHF admission. Our findings suggest that early reperfusion therapy leads to better clinical outcomes in terms of a composite of death/CHF even in patients with relatively delayed presentation (3 ≤ - <12 hours), although mortality benefit of early reperfusion is limited to about 3 hours after symptom onset. This result supports the indication of the current guideline for primary PCI, which recommend primary PCI for STEMI patients within 12 hours after symptom onset. Additionally, considering long-term efficacy of early reperfusion for patients who have already survived myocardial infarction, it is appropriate to evaluate not only death, but also a composite of death and CHF. Clearly, considering the risk of CHF is important to quality of life outcomes, and the composite endpoint of death/CHF may have a role as a clinical endpoint that reflects the long-term influence of infarction size in patients suffering from STEMI.

Regarding the influence of patient risk profile on the efficacy of early reperfusion by primary PCI, the magnitude of the impact of early reperfusion is greater in high-risk patients, although the tendency towards better outcomes was also observed in relatively low-risk patients. Thus, the absolute risk reduction due to a short O2B time was greater in high-risk patients such as those with CHF, anterior myocardial infarction and renal insufficiency, although the relative risk reduction was almost similar in high-risk patients and low-risk patients. This result shows a benefit of early reperfusion by primary PCI in all patients with STEMI, regardless of their risk profile.

Limitations

The current study has several limitations. First, we could not completely excluded the influence of patients' recall bias for symptom onset, of survivor bias and of variety in the time course of developing myocardial necrosis, as was also the case in previous studies. However, even if we consider that some patients did not reliably recall their symptom onset time, the result of the current analysis is meaningful in terms of triage and treatment of STEMI patients in daily clinical practice. Second, the huge differences in baseline characteristics between patients with early reperfusion and those with delayed reperfusion might limit the comparability of the groups, although we intended to adjust as extensively as possible to minimize the influence of unmeasured confounders. Finally, selection bias and residual confounding were inevitable in this type of observational study.

Conclusions

Despite these limitations, we conclude that having a symptom-onset-to-balloon (O2B) time of within 3 hours is associated with a lower long-term mortality rate in patients with STEMI who were treated with primary PCI and that the benefit of early reperfusion by primary PCI is present regardless of the risk profile of the patients.

不必要である．

これは主たる結果ではないので削除する．

References（省略）

Figure legends

Figure 1: Selection of study population

Figure 2: Relationship of symptom-onset-to-balloon (O2B) time with clinical outcomes

Figure 3: Relationship of door-to-balloon (D2B) time with clinical outcomes

Figure 4: Unadjusted Kaplan-Meier curves for cumulative incidence of a composite of death/CHF stratified by patient risk profile

Figure 5: Relative risk reduction of symptom-onset-to-balloon (O2B) time stratified by risk profile

Figure 1

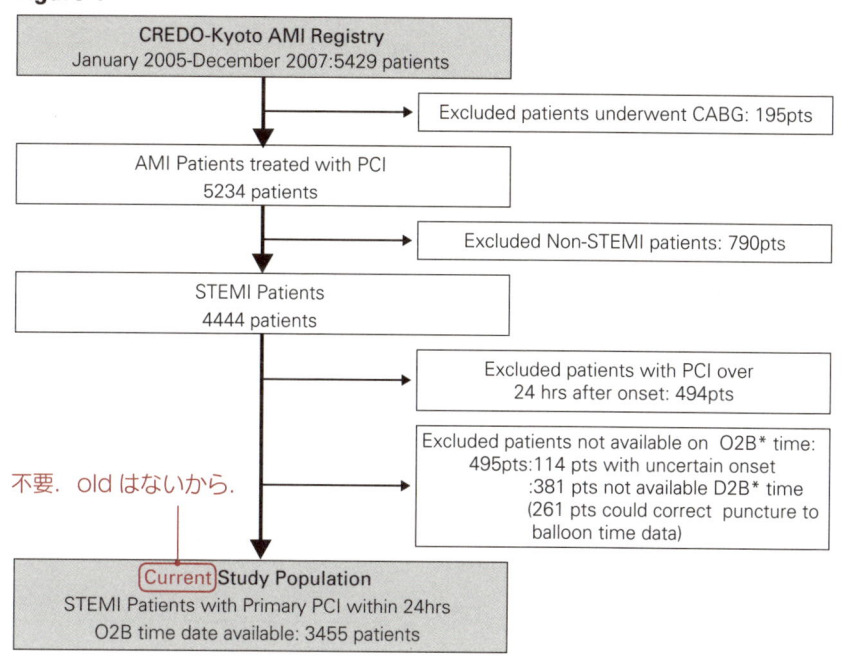

```
CREDO-Kyoto AMI Registry
January 2005-December 2007:5429 patients
                │
                ├──────────► Excluded patients underwent CABG: 195pts
                ▼
AMI Patients treated with PCI
5234 patients
                │
                ├──────────► Excluded Non-STEMI patients: 790pts
                ▼
STEMI Patients
4444 patients
                │
                ├──────────► Excluded patients with PCI over
                │            24 hrs after onset: 494pts
                │
                ├──────────► Excluded patients not available on O2B* time:
                │            495pts:114 pts with uncertain onset
                │            :381 pts not available D2B* time
                │            (261 pts could correct puncture to
                │            balloon time data)
                ▼
[Current] Study Population
STEMI Patients with Primary PCI within 24hrs
O2B time date available: 3455 patients
```

不要. old はないから.

Figure 2

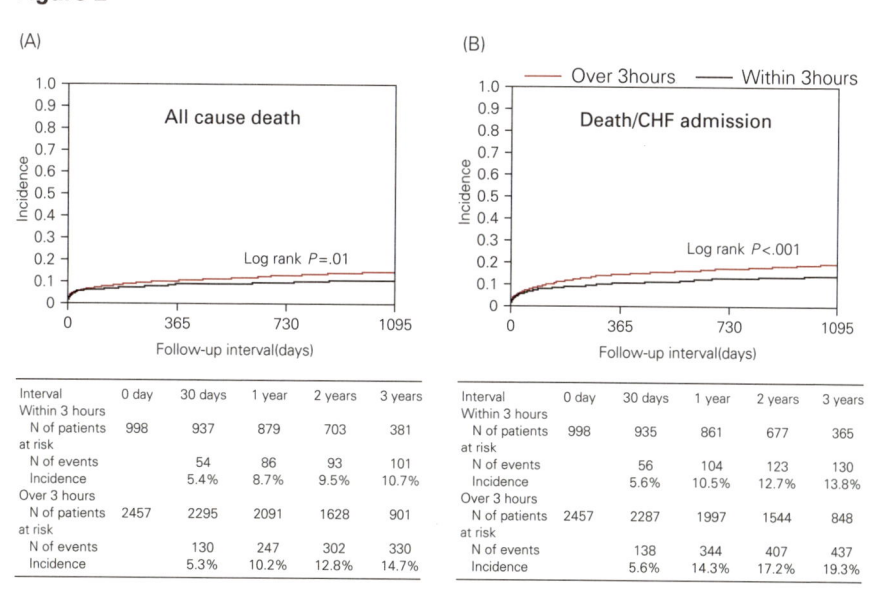

(A) All cause death — Log rank $P=.01$

(B) Death/CHF admission — Log rank $P<.001$ — Over 3hours / Within 3hours

Interval	0 day	30 days	1 year	2 years	3 years
Within 3 hours					
N of patients at risk	998	937	879	703	381
N of events		54	86	93	101
Incidence		5.4%	8.7%	9.5%	10.7%
Over 3 hours					
N of patients at risk	2457	2295	2091	1628	901
N of events		130	247	302	330
Incidence		5.3%	10.2%	12.8%	14.7%

Interval	0 day	30 days	1 year	2 years	3 years
Within 3 hours					
N of patients at risk	998	935	861	677	365
N of events		56	104	123	130
Incidence		5.6%	10.5%	12.7%	13.8%
Over 3 hours					
N of patients at risk	2457	2287	1997	1544	848
N of events		138	344	407	437
Incidence		5.6%	14.3%	17.2%	19.3%

3編　受動態より能動態を使う／％は分子分母も併記する

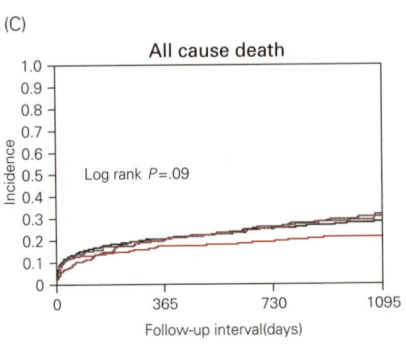

	1 — Within 3h	3 — 6h-12h
	2 — 3h-6h	4 — 12h-24h

(C) All cause death

Log rank *P*=.09

Interval	30 days	1 year	2 years	3 years
Within 3hours				
N of patients at risk 998	937	879	703	381
Incidence	5.4%	8.7%	9.5%	10.7%
3h～6h				
N of patients at risk 1377	1284	1180	934	523
Incidence	5.8%	10.2%	12.6%	14.1%
6h～12h				
N of patients at risk 667	621	570	435	241
Incidence	5.4%	10.4%	13.1%	15.7%
12h～24h				
N of patients at risk 413	390	343	259	137
Incidence	3.4%	9.8%	12.9%	15.2%

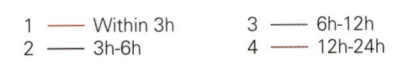

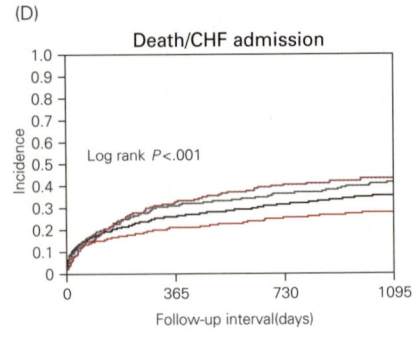

(D) Death/CHF admission

Log rank *P*<.001

Interval	30 days	1 year	2 years	3 years
Within 3hours				
N of patients at risk 998	935	861	677	365
Incidence	5.6%	10.5%	12.7%	13.8%
3h～6h				
N of patients at risk 1377	1279	1141	899	497
Incidence	6.2%	13.1%	15.8%	17.8%
6h～12h				
N of patients at risk 667	621	537	406	225
Incidence	5.4%	15.5%	18.2%	20.9%
12h～24h				
N of patients at risk 413	387	319	239	126
Incidence	4.2%	16.4%	20.3%	21.6%

Figure 3

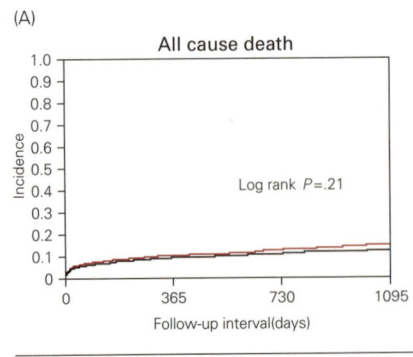

— >D2B 90min
— ≦D2B 90min

(A) All cause death

Log rank *P*=.21

Interval	0 day	30 days	1 year	2 years	3 years
>90min					
N of patients at risk	1671	1561	1427	1121	634
Incidence		5.4%	10.0%	12.5%	14.4%
≦90min					
N of patients at risk	1720	1618	1493	1169	622
Incidence		4.8%	9.2%	10.8%	12.4%

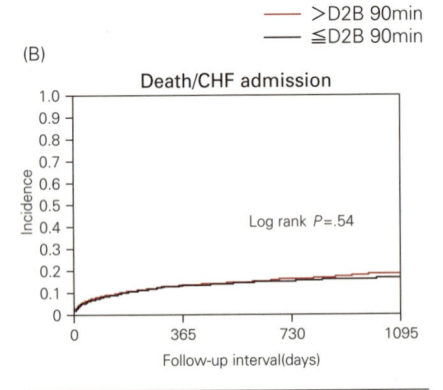

(B) Death/CHF admission

Log rank *P*=.54

Interval	0 day	30 days	1 year	2 years	3 years
>90min					
N of patients at risk	1671	1557	1378	1073	603
Incidence		5.6%	13.1%	16.2%	18.4%
≦90min					
N of patients at risk	1720	1612	1430	1108	585
Incidence		5.2%	13.1%	15.3%	16.7%

Before

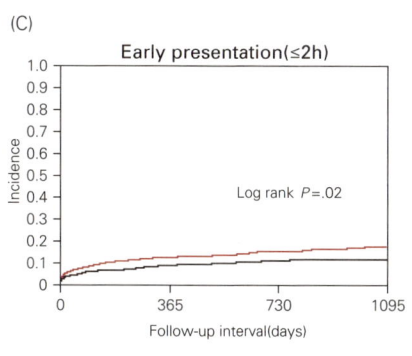

(C) Early presentation(≤2h)

Log rank *P*=.02

Interval	0 day	30 days	1 year	2 years	3 years
>90min					
N of patients at risk	719	668	598	486	270
Incidence		6.1%	12.8%	15.5%	17.7%
≤90min					
N of patients at risk	653	621	571	439	238
Incidence		4.3%	9.2%	11.0%	11.9%

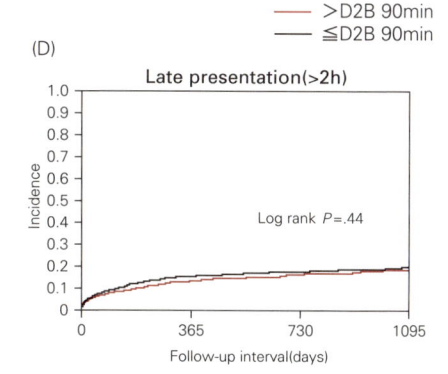

(D) Late presentation(>2h)

— >D2B 90min
— ≤D2B 90min

Log rank *P*=.44

Interval	0 day	30 days	1 year	2 years	3 years
>90min					
N of patients at risk	788	733	638	483	287
Incidence		5.4%	13.7%	16.8%	18.7%
≤90min					
N of patients at risk	1065	989	857	667	347
Incidence		5.8%	15.5%	17.9%	19.7%

Figure 4

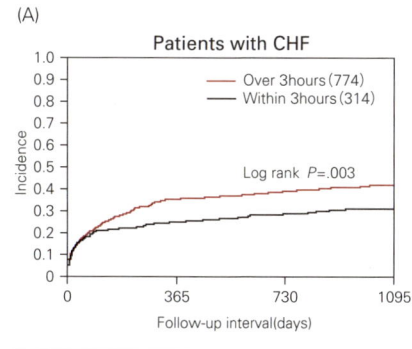

(A) Patients with CHF

— Over 3hours (774)
— Within 3hours (314)

Log rank *P*=.003

Interval	0 day	30 days	1 year	2 years	3 years
Within 3 hours					
N of patients at risk	314	263	226	177	106
Incidence		15.6%	25.1%	29.0%	30.9%
Over 3 hours					
N of patients at risk	774	620	448	330	175
Incidence		14.9%	35.4%	39.2%	42.4%

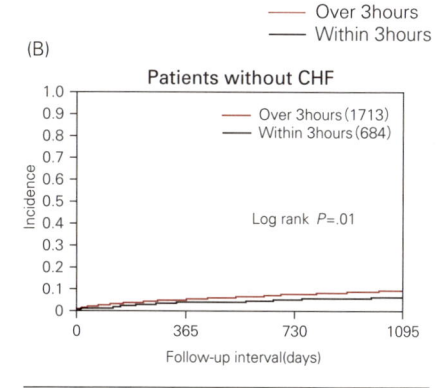

(B) Patients without CHF

— Over 3hours
— Within 3hours

— Over 3hours (1713)
— Within 3hours (684)

Log rank *P*=.01

Interval	0 day	30 days	1 year	2 years	3 years
Within 3 hours					
N of patients at risk	684	672	635	500	259
Incidence		1.0%	3.9%	5.2%	5.9%
Over 3 hours					
N of patients at risk	1713	1667	1549	1214	673
Incidence		1.6%	5.3%	7.8%	9.4%

3編 受動態より能動態を使う／％は分子分母も併記する

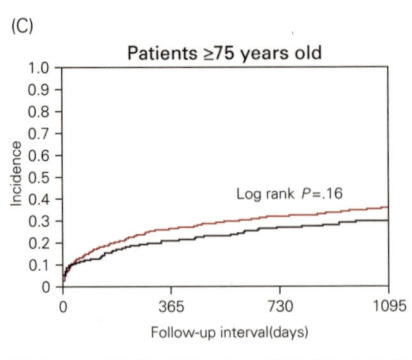

(C) Patients ≥75 years old

Log rank $P=.16$

Interval	0 day	30 days	1 year	2 years	3 years
Within 3 hours					
N of patients at risk	234	206	175	124	71
Incidence		10.7%	21.3%	27.2%	30.1%
Over 3 hours					
N of patients at risk	823	731	557	401	207
Incidence		10.1%	26.4%	32.2%	35.9%

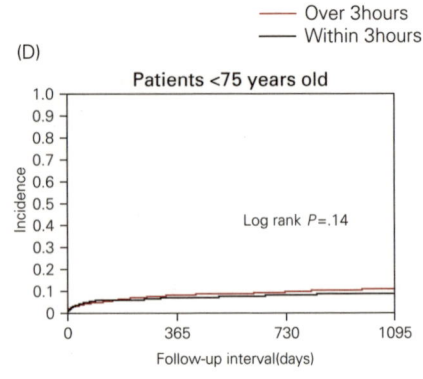

(D) Patients <75 years old

Log rank $P=.14$

Interval	0 day	30 days	1 year	2 years	3 years
Within 3 hours					
N of patients at risk	764	729	686	553	294
Incidence		4.1%	7.3%	8.3%	8.8%
Over 3 hours					
N of patients at risk	1634	1556	1440	1143	641
Incidence		3.4%	8.3%	9.8%	11.2%

— Over 3hours
— Within 3hours

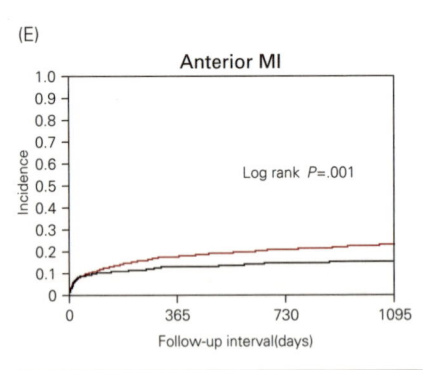

(E) Anterior MI

Log rank $P=.001$

Interval	0 day	30 days	1 year	2 years	3 years
Within 3 hours					
N of patients at risk	477	434	393	303	172
Incidence		8.4%	13.6%	14.8%	15.4%
Over 3 hours					
N of patients at risk	1160	1048	895	682	342
Incidence		8.1%	18.0%	21.3%	23.3%

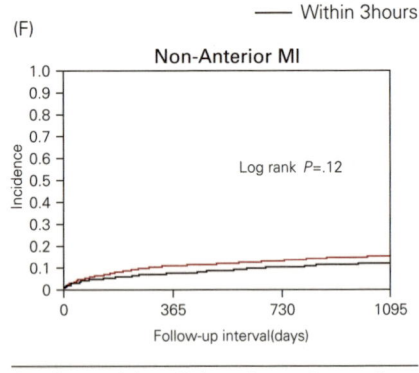

(F) Non-Anterior MI

Log rank $P=.12$

Interval	0 day	30 days	1 year	2 years	3 years
Within 3 hours					
N of patients at risk	521	501	468	374	193
Incidence		3.1%	7.8%	10.7%	12.2%
Over 3 hours					
N of patients at risk	1297	1239	1102	862	506
Incidence		3.5%	11.0%	13.5%	15.7%

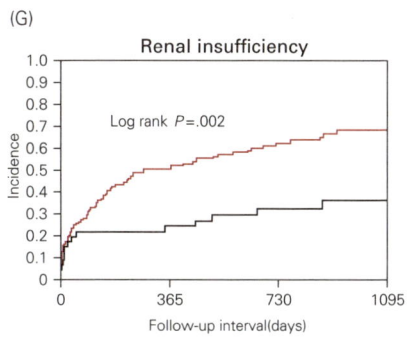

Before

(G) Renal insufficiency

Log rank *P*=.002

Interval	0 day	30 days	1 year	2 years	3 years
Within 3 hours					
N of patients at risk	46	38	30	20	10
Incidence		17.4%	24.3%	32.0%	36.3%
Over 3 hours					
N of patients at risk	135	104	61	33	10
Incidence		20.1%	50.4%	62.4%	68.4%

(H) Non-renal insufficiency

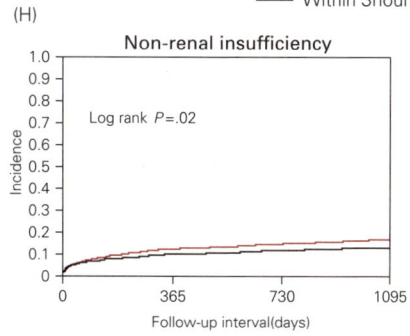

Log rank *P*=.02

Interval	0 day	30 days	1 year	2 years	3 years
Within 3 hours					
N of patients at risk	952	897	831	657	355
Incidence		5.1%	9.9%	11.7%	12.7%
Over 3 hours					
N of patients at risk	2322	2183	1936	1511	838
Incidence		4.8%	12.3%	14.7%	16.6%

(I) Multi vessel disease

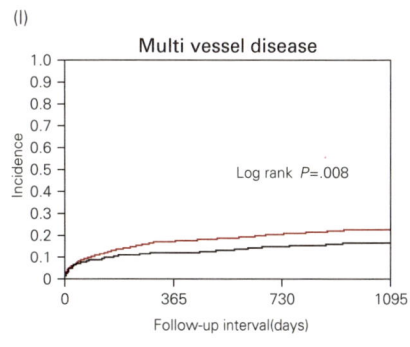

Log rank *P*=.008

Interval	0 day	30 days	1 year	2 years	3 years
Within 3 hours					
N of patients at risk	476	441	402	310	173
Incidence		6.7%	12.3%	15.2%	16.9%
Over 3 hours					
N of patients at risk	1276	1181	999	762	420
Incidence		6.5%	17.4%	20.8%	23.0%

(J) Single vessel disease

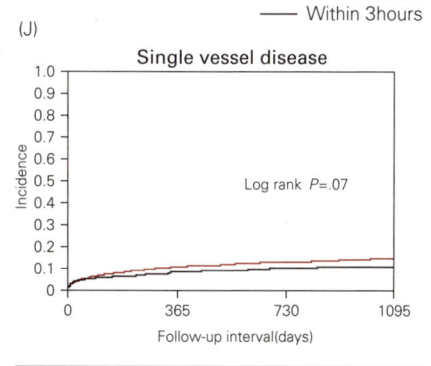

Log rank *P*=.07

Interval	0 day	30 days	1 year	2 years	3 years
Within 3 hours					
N of patients at risk	522	494	459	367	192
Incidence		4.6%	8.9%	10.4%	10.9%
Over 3 hours					
N of patients at risk	1181	1106	998	782	428
Incidence		4.7%	11.0%	13.3%	15.3%

3 編　受動態より能動態を使う／％は分子分母も併記する

Figure 5

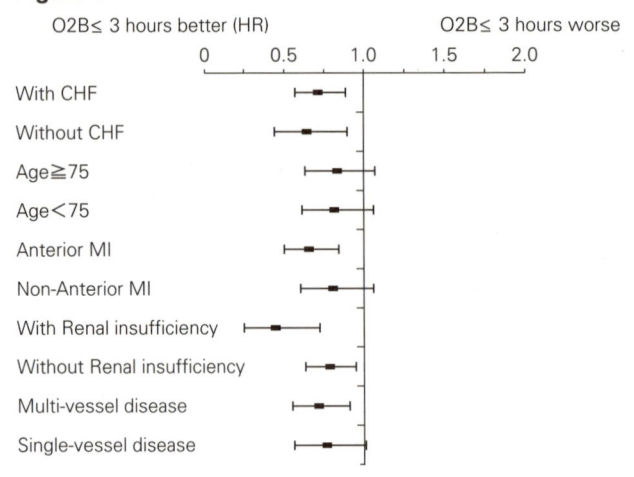

```
            O2B≤ 3 hours better (HR)        O2B≤ 3 hours worse
            0        0.5       1.0      1.5       2.0
With CHF                      ├─■─┤
Without CHF                   ├─■─┤
Age≧75                         ├─■─┤
Age＜75                        ├─■─┤
Anterior MI                    ├─■─┤
Non-Anterior MI                 ├■┤
With Renal insufficiency         ├──■──┤
Without Renal insufficiency     ├─■─┤
Multi-vessel disease           ├─■─┤
Single-vessel disease         ├───■───┤
```

Table 1 Baseline charactaristics[a]

Variables	Entire cohort (n =3455)	OTB time ≦3hours (n = 998)	OTB time ＞3 hours (n = 2457)	P value
Age, mean (SD), y	67.4 (12.2)	65.3 (12.0)	68.4 (12.2)	＜.001
≥75	1057 (31)	234 (23)	823 (34)	＜.001
Male	2556 (74)	794 (80)	1762 (72)	＜.001
BMI*, mean (SD)	23.6 (3.4)	23.8 (3.4)	23.4 (3.4)	.003
＜ 25.0	2496 (72)	707 (71)	1789 (73)	.24
Hypertension	2707 (78)	771 (77)	1936 (79)	.32
Diabetes mellitus	1085 (31)	322 (32)	763 (31)	.49
on insulin therapy	148 (4.3)	42 (4.2)	106 (4.3)	.89
on oral hypoglycemic agents	660 (19)	192 (19)	468 (19)	.90
History of smoking	2100 (61)	667 (67)	1433 (58)	＜.001
Current smoking	1406 (41)	459 (46)	947 (39)	＜.001
Heart failure	1075(31%)	317(32%)	758(31%)	.60
Ejection fraction, mean (SD)	52.5 (12.7)	53.6 (12.9)	52.1 (12.6)	.006
≤ 40%	451 (17)	122 (15)	329 (18)	.14
Prior myocardial infarction	298 (8.6)	103 (10)	195 (7.9)	.03
Prior Stroke (symptomatic)	292 (8.5)	67 (6.7)	225 (9.2)	.02
Peripheral vascular disease	104 (3.0)	26 (2.6)	78 (3.2)	.37
eGFR (mL/min/1.73m^2)[b]*, median (IQR)	69.4 (54.1-85.4)	68.2 (53.3-82.2)	70.2 (54.4-86.3)	.04
eGFR ＜30,without hemodialysis	136 (3.9)	33 (3.3)	103 (4.2)	.22
Hemodialysis	45 (1.3)	13 (1.3)	32 (1.3)	.99
Atrial fibrillation	320 (9.3)	102 (10)	218 (8.9)	.22

このデータは skew するので
このまま median(IQR) でよい．

下に Current があって History の意
味するところがわかりにくいので，
下の Current のみでよい．

Before

Anemia (Hb <11.0g/dl)	318 (9.2)	67 (6.7)	251 (10.2)	<.001
Thrombocytopenia (PLT<10*104)	58 (1.7)	22 (2.2)	36 (1.5)	.14
COPD	108 (3.1)	28 (2.8)	80 (3.3)	.49
Liver chirrosis	76 (2.2)	22 (2.2)	54 (2.2)	.99
Malignancy	262 (7.6)	69 (6.9)	193 (7.9)	.34
Presentation				
Hours from onset to presentation*, median (IQR)	2.6 (1.3-5.5)	1.0 (0.7-1.4)	3.7 (2.3-7.5)	<.001
Hours from onset to balloon*, median (IQR)	4.2 (2.8-7.3)	2.3 (1.9-2.7)	5.5 (4.0-9.4)	<.001
< 3 hours	998 (29)	998 (100)	0 (0)	
3-6 hours	1377 (40)		1377 (56)	<.001
6-12 hours	667 (19)		667 (27)	
12-24 hours	413 (12)		413 (17)	
Hours from door to balloon*, median (IQR)	1.5 (1.0-2.2)	1.3 (0.9-1.7)	1.7 (1.1-2.5)	0.9
<= 90 minutes	1621 (54)	635 (66)	1085 (45)	<.001
Hemodynamics				
Killip class 1	2593 (75)	722 (72)	1871 (76)	
Killip class 2	292 (8.5)	70 (7.0)	222 (9.0)	<.001
Killip class 3	87 (2.5)	19 (1.9)	68 (2.8)	
Killip class 4	483 (14)	187 (19)	296 (12)	
Cardiac arrest	103 (3.0)	46 (4.6)	57 (2.3)	<.001
Cardiogenic shock at presentation	483 (14)	187 (19)	296 (12)	<.001
Disturbance of consciousness	299 (8.7)	113 (11)	186 (7.6)	<.001
Intubation	187 (5.4)	61 (6.1)	126 (5.1)	.25
IABP use	549 (16)	181 (18)	368 (15)	.02
PCPS use	98 (2.8)	40 (4.0)	58 (2.4)	.01
Mechanical complications				
Ventricular septal perforation	6 (0.2)	2 (0.2)	4 (0.2)	.99
Severe mitral regurgitation	17 (0.5)	7 (0.7)	10 (0.4)	.29
Right ventricular infarction	71 (2.1)	26 (2.6)	45 (1.8)	.16
Free wall rupture	24 (0.7)	5 (0.5)	19 (0.8)	.37
AV block	202 (5.8)	81 (8.1)	121 (4.9)	<.001
Ventricular tachycardia	383 (11)	126 (13)	257 (10)	.07
Ventricular fibrillation	220 (6.4)	79 (7.9)	141 (5.7)	.02

Abbreviations: SD, standard deviation; BMI, body mass index, calculated as weight in kilograms divided by height in meters squared;
  eGFR, estimated glomerular filtration rate; IQR, interquartile range; Hb, hemogrobin; PLT, platelet;
  COPD, chronic obstructive pulmonary disease; IABP, intraaortic balloon pumping; PCPS, percutaneous cardiopulmonary support
a Data are expressed as No. (%) unless otherwise indicated.
b eGFR calculated by the Modification of Diet in Renal Disease formula modified for Japanese patients13.
* Potential independent variables selected for Cox proportional hazard models.

本来０のはずなので０を埋める．

3編　受動態より能動態を使う／%は分子分母も併記する

Table 2 Angiographic characteristics

重要なのを選んで Table1 にくっつける.

Variables	Entire cohort	OTB time ≤3hours	OTB time >3 hours	p value
Infarct location				
Anterior	1637 (47)	477 (48)	1160 (47)	
Inferior	1407 (41)	429 (43)	978 (40)	.01
Posterior	305 (8.8)	69 (6.9)	236 (9.6)	
Lateral	106 (3.1)	23 (2.3)	83 (3.4)	
Infarct-related artery location				
LAD	1614 (47)	453 (45)	1161 (47)	
LCX	343 (10)	80 (8.0)	263 (11)	
RCA	1409 (41)	428 (43)	981 (40)	.004
LMCA	74 (2.1)	33 (3.3)	41 (1.7)	
CABG Graft	15 (0.4)	4 (0.4)	11 (0.5)	
Number of vessels diseased				
Single vessel disease	1639 (47)	496 (50)	1143 (47)	
Double vessel disease	1026 (30)	305 (31)	721 (29)	
Triple vessel disease	596 (17)	135 (14)	461 (19)	.01
LMCA disease	155 (4.5)	51 (5.1)	104 (4.2)	
Post CABG	39 (1.1)	11 (1.1)	28 (1.1)	
Multivessel disease*	1752 (51)	476 (48)	1276 (52)	.02
Multivessel/LMCA disease	1816 (53)	502 (50)	1314 (53)	.09
Involvement of proximal LAD	2268 (66)	634 (64)	1634 (67)	.10
Involvement of LAD	2470 (71)	689 (69)	1781 (72)	.043
Involvement of RCA	2015 (58)	576 (58)	1439 (59)	.65
Involvement of LCX	1340 (39)	340 (34)	1000 (41)	<.001
Involvemwnt of LMCA	162 (4.7)	52 (5.2)	110 (4.5)	.36
Presence of CTO	370 (11)	96 (9.6)	274 (11)	.18
Procedural characteristics				
Arterial access				
Femoral	2901 (84)	885 (89)	2016 (82)	
Radial	419 (12)	71 (7.1)	348 (14)	<.001
Brachial	119 (3.5)	38 (3.8)	81 (3.3)	
Arterial sheath, median (IQR), F	7 (6 - 7)	7 (6 - 7)	7 (6 - 7)	.03
Staged PCI	763 (22)	211 (21)	552 (22)	.39
Number of target vessels, median (IQR)	1 (1 - 2)	1 (1 - 2)	1 (1 - 2)	.34
mean (SD)	1.30 (0.54)	1.31 (0.55)	1.29 (0.54)	
Number of target lesions, median (IQR)	1 (1 - 2)	1 (1 - 2)	1 (1 - 2)	.73
mean (IQR)	1.39 (0.69)	1.38 (0.68)	1.39 (0.70)	
Target of proximal LAD*	1886 (55)	540 (54)	1346 (55)	.72
Target of LAD	1977 (57)	561 (56)	1416 (58)	.45
Target of RCA	1661 (48)	498 (50)	1163 (47)	.17

multivessel(≧ 2) をまとめる.

				Before
Target of LCX	660 (19)	166 (17)	494 (20)	.02
Target of unprotected LMCA*	112 (3.2)	48 (4.8)	64 (2.6)	.001
Target of CTO*	109 (3.2)	32 (3.2)	77 (3.1)	.91
Target of bifurcation*	897 (26)	258 (26)	639 (26)	.92
Side-branch stenting*	103 (3.0)	34 (3.4)	69 (2.8)	.35
Total number of stents, median (IQR)	1 (1 - 2)	1 (1 - 2)	1 (1 - 2)	.51
mean (SD)	1.67 (1.1)	1.65 (1.1)	1.67 (1.1)	
Total stent length (mm), median (IQR)	24 (18 - 42)	25 (18 - 42)	26 (18 - 42)	.83
mean (SD)	34.6 (24.5)	34.6 (24.7)	34.6 (24.5)	
Total stent length >28mm*	1333 (42)	393 (42)	940 (41)	.65
Minimum stent size (mm)	3 (2.5 - 3.5)	3 (2.75 - 3.5)	3 (2.5 - 3.5)	
	3.05 (0.46)	3.10 (0.47)	3.03 (0.46)	
Minimum stent size <3.0mm*	978 (31)	256 (28)	722 (32)	.02
DES use(culprit)*	596 (17)	155 (16)	411 (18)	.09
Thrombectomy*	2185 (63)	688 (69)	1497 (61)	<.001
Distal protection*	306 (8.9)	78 (7.8)	228 (9.3)	.17
Complications				
Side branch occlusion	163 (4.7)	35 (3.5)	128 (5.2)	.03
Coronary Dissection	37 (1.1)	8 (0.8)	29 (1.2)	.31
Thrombosis	21 (0.6)	8 (0.8)	13 (0.5)	.36
Slow flow	320 (9.2)	68 (6.8)	252 (10)	.001
Acute occlusion(transient)	49 (1.4)	16 (1.6)	33 (1.3)	.56
Acute occlusion (persistent)	11 (0.3)	1 (0.1)	10 (0.4)	.11
Coronary perforation	12 (0.3)	2 (0.2)	10 (0.4)	.32

Abbreviations: LAD, left anterior decending artery; LCX, left circumflex artery; RCA, right coronary artery; LMCA, left main coronary artery; CABG, coronary artery bypass graft surgery; CTO, chronic total occlusion; IQR, interquartile range; F, french; PCI, percutaneous coronary intervention; DES,drug eluting stent;

[a] Data are shown as No. (%) unless otherwise specified.

* Potential independent variables selected for Cox proportional hazard models.

3編　受動態より能動態を使う／％は分子分母も併記する

Table 3 Medications at discharge[a]

重要なのを選んで Table1 にくっつける.

Variables	Entire cohort	OTB time ≦3hours	OTB time >3 hours	p value
Antiplatelet therapy				
Thienopyridine	3312 (96)	957 (96)	2355 (96)	.95
Ticlopidine	3031 (92)	886 (93)	2145 (91)	.17
Clopidogrel	280 (8.5)	71 (7.4)	209 (8.9)	
Aspirin	3406 (99)	982 (98)	2424 (99)	.56
Cilostazole*	1286 (37)	330 (33)	956 (39)	.001
Other medications				
Statins*	1856 (54)	568 (57)	430 (43)	.02
Beta-blockers*	1416 (41)	438 (44)	978 (40)	.03
ACE-I/ARB*	2491 (72)	728 (73)	1763 (72)	.48
ACE-I	1189 (34)	366 (37)	823 (34)	.08
ARB	1370 (40)	387 (39)	983 (40)	
Nitrates*	1034 (30)	301 (30)	733 (30)	.85
Calcium chanel blockers*	661 (19)	194 (19)	467 (19)	.77
Nicolandil*	988 (29)	265 (27)	723 (29)	.09
Coumadin*	351 (10)	109 (11)	242 (9.9)	.35
Proton pump inhibitors*	1154 (33)	335 (34)	819 (33)	.90
H2-blockers*	1168 (34)	322 (32)	846 (34)	.22

Abbreviations: ACE-I, angiotensin converting enzyme inhibitor; ARB, angiotensin II receptor blocker;
a Data are shown as No. (%) unless otherwise specified.
* Potential independent variables selected for Cox proportional hazard models.

Table 4 Multivariate analysis for death/CHF (Cox propotional hazard model)

Variables	Univariate HR	(95% C.I)	p value	Multivariate HR	(95% C.I)	p value
OTB≦3hrs	0.76	0.61-0.94	.01	0.73	0.59-0.92	.007
DES（culprit DES use）	0.79	0.62-0.98	.03	0.75	0.53-1.07	.11
Aspiration	0.72	0.61-0.85	<.001	0.80	0.66-0.98	.03
Distal protection	0.78	0.56-1.06	.11	0.82	0.57-1.19	.29
Age >= 75 years	3.64	3.09-4.29	<.001	1.78	1.43-2.21	<.001
Male	0.6	0.50-0.71	<.001	0.84	0.68-1.04	.12
BMI <25.0	2.58	2.05-3.28	<.001	1.42	1.09-1.86	.01
Hypertension	0.78	0.65-0.94	.01	1.34	1.06-1.68	.01
Diabetes mellitus on insulin therapy	1.71	1.21-2.33	.003	1.01	0.70-1.45	.98
Current smoking	0.51	0.42-0.61	<.001	0.91	0.73-1.14	.40
Heart failure	6	5.04-7.14	<.001	3.16	2.51-3.98	<.001

Before

Shock at presentation	5.08	4.32-5.98	<.001	1.47	1.16-1.85	.001
Multivessel disease	1.58	1.34-1.86	<.001	1.50	1.22-1.83	<.001
Mitral regurgitation grade 3/4	2.89	2.03-3.99	<.001	1.10	0.73-1.65	.66
Prior myocardial infarction	1.77	1.39-2.22	<.001	1.62	1.22-2.14	<.001
Prior Stroke	2.02	1.60-2.53	<.001	1.29	0.99-1.69	.057
Peripheral vascular disease	2.51	1.77-3.46	<.001	1.33	0.89-1.98	.17
Dialysis	3.97	2.54-5.88	<.001	2.37	1.41-4.00	.001
eGFR <30, not on dialysis	5.21	4.06-6.60	<.001	1.55	1.13-2.12	.01
Atrial fibrillation	2.21	1.78-2.72	<.001	1.06	0.81-1.38	.68
Anemia (Hb <11.0g/dl)	3.47	2.84-4.19	<.001	1.18	0.92-1.51	.19
Platelet <100*109/L	4.42	3.03-6.20	<.001	2.74	1.76-4.28	<.001
COPD	1.3	0.83-1.92	0.24	1.04	0.64-1.69	.87
Liver cirrhosis	1.28	0.76-2.01	0.33	1.06	0.61-1.82	.84
Malignancy	2.46	1.96-3.05	<.001	1.71	1.32-2.22	<.001
Target of proximal LAD	1.09	0.92-1.28	0.31	1.30	1.05-1.60	.01
Target of unprotected LMCA	4.17	3.11-5.47	<.001	2.42	1.68-3.47	<.001
Target of CTO	1.53	1.01-2.22	.047	1.14	0.72-1.80	.57
Target of bifurcation	1.28	1.07-1.53	.007	1.23	0.98-1.54	.07
Side-branch stenting	1.41	0.91-2.07	.12	0.91	0.56-1.46	.69
Total stent length >28mm	0.98	0.82-1.17	.81	0.73	0.59-0.91	.005
Minimum stent size <3.0mm	1.17	0.97-1.40	.10	0.84	0.67-1.05	.13
Cilostazol	0.78	0.66-0.93	.004	0.88	0.67-1.17	.38
Statins	0.33	0.27-0.39	<.001	0.50	0.40-0.62	<.001
Beta-blockers	0.59	0.50-0.71	<.001	0.77	0.62-0.95	.01
ACE-I/ARB	0.31	0.26-0.36	<.001	0.47	0.38-0.57	<.001
Nitrates	0.69	0.57-0.83	<.001	0.58	0.45-0.74	<.001
Calcium chanel blockers	0.75	0.60-0.93	0.01	0.74	0.57-0.95	.02
Nicorandil	0.69	0.57-0.83	<.001	1.00	0.79-1.27	.98
Coumadin	1.04	0.80-1.34	.75	0.85	0.62-1.17	.32
Proton pump inhibitors	1.00	0.85-1.19	.96	0.72	0.58-0.89	.003
H2-blockers	0.55	0.46-0.67	<.001	0.64	0.50-0.81	<.001

Abbreviations: HR, hazard ratio; CI, confidence interval; O2B, onset to balloon; DES, drug eluting stent; eGFR, estimated glomerular filtration rate; Hb, hemogrobin; COPD, chronic obstructive pulmonary disease; LAD, left anterior decending artery; LMCA, left main coronary artery; CTO, chronic total occlusion; ACE-I, angiotensin converting enzyme inhibitor; ARB, angiotensin Ⅱ receptor blocker

リスクファクター論文ではなくonset-to-balloon時間が予後に与える影響をみるので一番上のonset-to-balloon時間のadjusted HRだけでよくtextに変更.

Table 5 Multivariate analysis for death/CHF (Cox propotional hazard model)

	Early presentation (≤ 2 hours)						Delayed presentation (> 2 hours)					
	Univariate			Multivariate			Univariate			Multivariate		
Variables	HR	95% C.I	p value	HR	95% C.I	p value	HR	95% C.I	p value	HR	95% C.I	p value
D2B≤90 min	0.72	0.54-0.95	.02	0.54	0.35-0.85	.008	1.09	0.88-1.35	.44	1.57	1.12-2.18	.008
DES（culprit DES use）	0.57	0.36-0.87	.008	0.50	0.24-1.04	.06	0.84	0.61-1.13	.25	0.81	0.51-1.29	.38
Thrombectomy	0.74	0.56-0.99	.04	0.64	0.44-0.92	.02	0.80	0.65-0.99	.04	0.90	0.69-1.16	.40
Distal protection	0.67	0.32-1.23	.21	0.69	0.30-1.62	.40	0.81	0.55-1.15	.25	0.87	0.56-1.35	.53
Age >= 75 years	3.32	2.51-4.37	<.001	1.88	1.25-2.82	.002	3.56	2.87-4.44	<.001	1.88	1.40-2.51	<.001
Male	0.59	0.44-0.80	<.001	0.71	0.46-1.08	.11	0.62	0.50-0.77	<.001	0.86	0.65-1.14	.29
BMI <25.0	2.22	1.55-3.30	<.001	1.18	0.74-1.88	.49	2.72	2.02-3.76	<.001	1.44	1.01-2.05	.043
Hypertension	0.66	0.49-0.90	.009	1.55	1.007-2.38	.047	0.81	0.64-1.05	.10	1.20	0.88-1.62	.25
Diabetes mellitus on insulin therapy	1.62	0.88-2.73	.12	0.87	0.42-1.80	.71	1.45	0.88-2.24	.13	0.94	0.56-1.59	.82
Current smoking	0.61	0.45-0.81	<.001	0.90	0.60-1.36	.62	0.46	0.36-0.58	<.001	0.80	0.59-1.07	.13
Heart failure	6.07	4.51-8.27	<.001	2.84	1.76-4.60	<.001	5.82	4.66-7.30	<.001	3.37	2.52-4.50	<.001
Shock at presentation	5.17	3.91-6.82	<.001	1.99	1.22-3.23	.006	4.50	3.53-5.68	<.001	1.19	0.87-1.63	.28
Multivessel disease	1.55	1.17-2.06	.002	1.32	0.89-1.94	.17	1.54	1.24-1.91	<.001	1.70	1.29-2.23	<.001
Mitral regurgitation grade 3/4	4.41	2.58-7.03	<.001	1.48	0.71-3.08	.30	1.96	1.09-3.21	.03	0.72	0.38-1.34	.30
Prior myocardial infarction	1.37	0.90-2.00	.14	1.11	0.65-1.88	.70	1.88	1.33-2.58	<.001	2.15	1.45-3.17	<.001
Prior Stroke	1.87	1.19-2.80	.008	1.68	1.01-2.80	.045	2.00	1.48-2.65	<.001	1.15	0.79-1.66	.47
Peripheral vascular disease	2.42	1.24-4.23	.01	1.96	0.75-5.10	.17	2.18	1.36-3.31	.002	1.27	0.73-2.18	.40
Dialysis	4.35	1.96-8.25	<.001	3.88	1.52-9.88	.005	3.55	1.83-6.16	<.001	2.06	0.88-4.80	.10
eGFR <30, not on dialysis	4.37	2.66-6.76	<.001	2.11	1.06-4.19	.03	5.71	4.16-7.67	<.001	1.62	1.08-2.43	.02
Atrial fibrillation	1.97	1.34-2.82	.001	1.18	0.72-1.95	.51	2.50	1.88-3.27	<.001	1.09	0.77-1.54	.64
Anemia (Hb <11.0g/dl)	3.56	2.44-5.04	<.001	0.98	0.57-1.66	.93	3.10	2.39-3.96	<.001	1.20	0.86-1.69	.29

Platelet <100*10⁹/L	4.98	2.82-8.15	<.001	2.58	1.15-5.81	.02	4.32	2.46-6.98	<.001	3.15	1.65-5.99	<.001
COPD	1.07	0.46-2.11	.85	0.83	0.31-2.20	.70	1.47	0.84-2.37	.17	0.98	0.53-1.81	.94
Liver cirrhosis	1.42	0.60-2.79	.39	0.95	0.34-2.68	.92	1.22	0.58-2.22	.57	1.22	0.57-2.60	.61
Malignancy	2.76	1.87-3.96	<.001	2.16	1.27-3.65	.004	2.26	1.66-3.01	<.001	1.57	1.11-2.22	.01
Target of proximal LAD	0.80	0.61-1.05	.11	1.19	0.79-1.78	.41	1.29	1.04-1.61	.02	1.27	0.97-1.67	.08
Target of unprotected LMCA	6.33	4.20-9.20	<.001	2.92	1.63-5.21	<.001	2.74	1.67-4.23	<.001	1.91	1.07-3.40	.03
Target of CTO	2.23	1.17-3.81	.02	1.52	0.72-3.21	.27	1.33	0.72-2.21	.34	0.77	0.39-1.51	.45
Target of bifurcation	1.74	1.30-2.32	<.001	1.90	1.26-2.87	.002	1.04	0.81-1.31	.77	1.02	0.75-1.39	.90
Side-branch stenting	1.81	0.86-3.33	.11	0.60	0.26-1.39	.23	1.05	0.54-1.83	.86	1.18	0.59-2.35	.65
Total stent length >28mm	1.07	0.79-1.44	.66	0.70	0.47-1.05	.08	0.94	0.75-1.18	.61	0.76	0.57-1.02	.07
Minimum stent size <3.0mm	1.51	1.10-2.06	.01	1.25	0.82-1.91	.30	0.97	0.76-1.22	.77	0.63	0.46-0.85	.002
Cilostazol	0.69	0.50-0.93	.02	0.58	0.35-0.98	.04	0.89	0.71-1.11	.29	1.21	0.83-1.76	.31
Statins	0.29	0.21-0.38	<.001	0.45	0.30-0.68	<.001	0.37	0.30-0.47	<.001	0.50	0.38-0.66	<.001
Beta-blockers	0.54	0.40-0.73	<.001	0.74	0.50-1.12	.16	0.69	0.54-0.86	.001	0.87	0.66-1.15	.33
ACE-I/ARB	0.25	0.19-0.32	<.001	0.36	0.24-0.54	<.001	0.36	0.29-0.45	<.001	0.53	0.41-0.69	<.001
Nitrates	0.68	0.47-0.94	.02	0.58	0.35-0.97	.04	0.70	0.55-0.89	.003	0.52	0.38-0.72	<.001
Calcium chanel blockers	0.66	0.44-0.96	.03	0.72	0.45-1.18	.19	0.75	0.55-1.006	.055	0.60	0.42-0.85	.004
Nicorandil	0.74	0.54-1.01	.06	0.73	0.47-1.13	.16	0.78	0.60-0.99	.04	1.05	0.77-1.44	.76
Coumadin	0.87	0.53-1.35	.55	0.55	0.28-1.10	.09	1.29	0.91-1.77	.14	1.10	0.73-1.64	.66
Proton pump inhibitors	0.98	0.72-1.32	.90	0.81	0.53-1.23	.32	0.97	0.77-1.21	.78	0.68	0.51-0.91	.01
H2-blockers	0.55	0.39-0.76	<.001	0.71	0.46-1.09	.11	0.59	0.46-0.75	<.001	0.60	0.43-0.82	.001

Abbreviations: HR, hazard ratio; CI, confidence interval; D2B, door to balloon; DES, drug eluting stent; eGFR, estimated glomerular filtration rate; Hb, hemogrobin; COPD, chronic obstructive pulmonary disease; LAD, left anterior decending artery; LMCA, left main coronary artery; CTO, chronic total occlusion; ACE-I, angiotensin converting enzyme inhibitor; ARB, angiotensin Ⅱ receptor blocker

3編　受動態より能動態を使う／％は分子分母も併記する

After

このBMJのように，雑誌によっては，編集者がかなりの裁量権をもって論文構成を変えることがある．

RESEARCH

Association of onset to balloon and door to balloon time with long term clinical outcome in patients with ST elevation acute myocardial infarction having primary percutaneous coronary intervention: observational study

OPEN ACCESS

Hiroki Shiomi *MD/PhD candidate*[1], Yoshihisa Nakagawa *director*[2], Takeshi Morimoto *professor*[3], Yutaka Furukawa *director*[4], Akira Nakano *associate professor*[5], Shinichi Shirai *cardiologist*[6], Ryoji Taniguchi *cardiologist*[7], Kyohei Yamaji *cardiologist*[6], Kazuya Nagao *cardiologist*[8], Tamaki Suyama *cardiologist*[9], Hirokazu Mitsuoka *cardiologist*[10], Makoto Araki *cardiologist*[11], Hiroyuki Takashima *assistant professor*[12], Tetsu Mizoguchi *cardiologist*[13], Hiroshi Eisawa *director*[14], Seigo Sugiyama *associate professor*[15], Takeshi Kimura *professor*[1], on behalf of the CREDO-Kyoto AMI investigators

[1]Department of Cardiovascular Medicine, Graduate School of Medicine, Kyoto University, Kyoto, 606-8507, Japan; [2]Division of Cardiology, Tenri Hospital, 200 Mishimacho, Tenri city, Nara, 632-8552, Japan; [3]Center for General Internal Medicine and Emergency Care, Kinki University School of Medicine, Sayama-city, Osaka 589-8511, Japan; [4]Division of Cardiology, Kobe City Medical Center General Hospital, Chuo-ku, Kobe, 650-0046, Japan; [5]Division of Cardiology, University of Fukui Hospital, Yoshidagun, Fukui, 910-1193, Japan; [6]Division of Cardiology, Kokura Memorial Hospital, Kitakyushu, Fukuoka, 802-8555, Japan; [7]Division of Cardiology, Hyogo Prefectural Amagasaki Hospital, Amagasaki, Hyogo, 660-0828, Japan; [8]Division of Cardiology, Osaka Red Cross Hospital, Tennoji-ku, Osaka, 543-8555, Japan; [9]Division of Cardiology, Sapporo Higashi Tokushukai Hospital, Higashi-ku, Sapporo, 065-0033, Japan; [10]Division of Cardiology, Kishiwada City Hospital, Kishiwada, Osaka, 596-8501, Japan; [11]Division of Cardiology, Shimada Municipal Hospital, Shimada, Shizuoka 427-8502, Japan; [12]Department of Cardiovascular and Respiratory Medicine, Shiga University of Medical Science Hospital, Ostu, Shiga, 520-2192, Japan; [13]Division of Cardiology, Mitsubishi Kyoto Hospital, Nishigyo-ku Kyoto, 615-8087, Japan; [14]Division of Cardiology, Nishi-Kobe Medical Center, Nishi-ku, Kobe, 651-2273, Japan; [15]Department of Cardiovascular Medicine, Graduate School of Medical Sciences, Kumamoto University, Honjo, Kumamoto, 860-8556, Japan

Abstract

Objective To evaluate the relation of symptom onset to balloon time and door to balloon time with long term clinical outcome in patients with ST segment elevation myocardial infarction (STEMI) having primary percutaneous coronary intervention.

Design Observation of large cohort of patients with acute myocardial infarction.

Setting 26 tertiary hospitals in Japan.

Participants 3391 patients with STEMI who had primary percutaneous coronary intervention within 24 hours of symptom onset.

Main outcome measures Composite of death and congestive heart failure, compared by onset to balloon time and door to balloon time.

Results Compared with an onset to balloon time greater than 3 hours, a time of less than 3 hours was associated with a lower incidence of a composite of death and congestive heart failure (13.5% (123/964) *v* 19.2% (429/2427), P<0.001; relative risk reduction 29.7%). After adjustment for confounders, a short onset to balloon time was independently associated with a lower risk of the composite endpoint (adjusted hazard ratio 0.70, 95% confidence interval 0.56 to 0.88; P=0.002). However, no significant difference was found in the incidence of a composite of death and congestive heart failure between the two groups of patients with short (≤90 minutes) and long (>90 minutes) door to balloon time (16.7% (270/1671) *v* 18.4% (282/1720), P=0.54; relative risk reduction 9.2%). After adjustment for confounders, no significant difference was seen in the risk of the composite endpoint between the two groups of patients with short and long door to balloon time (adjusted hazard ratio: 0.98, 0.78 to 1.24: P=0.87). A door to balloon time of less than 90 minutes was associated with a lower incidence of a composite of death and congestive heart failure in patients who presented within 2 hours of symptom onset (11.9% (74/883) v 18.1% (147/655), P=0.01; relative risk reduction 34.3%) but not in patients who presented later (19.7% (196/788) v 18.7% (135/1065), P=0.44; −5.3%). Short door to balloon time was independently associated with a lower risk of a composite of death and congestive heart failure in patients with early presentation (adjusted hazard ratio 0.58, 0.38 to 0.87; P=0.009) but not in patients with delayed presentation (1.57, 1.12 to 2.18; P=0.008). A significant interaction was seen between door to balloon time and time to presentation (interaction P=0.01).

Conclusions Short onset to balloon time was associated with better 3 year clinical outcome in patients with STEMI having primary percutaneous coronary intervention, whereas the benefit of short door to balloon time was limited to patients who presented early. Efforts to minimise onset to balloon time, including reduction of patient related delay, should be recommended to improve clinical outcome in STEMI patients.

Introduction

Primary percutaneous coronary intervention is considered to play a central role in the treatment of ST segment elevation myocardial infarction (STEMI).[1 2] The American College of Cardiology/American Heart Association guideline for STEMI recommends primary percutaneous coronary intervention within 90 minutes of first medical contact, or door to balloon time, as a class 1 recommendation and also recommends a total ischaemic time within 120 minutes.[3 4] The European Society of Cardiology guideline for STEMI recommends primary percutaneous coronary intervention within 120 minutes of first medical contact in all cases and within 90 minutes in patients presenting early (less than two hours) with a large infarct and low risk of bleeding.[5] However, reports from previous studies are inconsistent regarding the effect of onset to balloon and door to balloon times on clinical outcomes in patients with STEMI having primary percutaneous coronary intervention.[6-9] Several relatively small studies suggested a positive correlation between short onset to balloon time and decreased mortality,[8 9] whereas the largest study, which enrolled more than 20 000 patients (national registry of myocardial infarction in the United States), found that in-hospital mortality did not increase with increasing delay in onset to balloon time.[6 7] Furthermore, short door to balloon time was associated with lower in-hospital mortality regardless of time from symptom onset to presentation in the US study,[6 7] whereas several other registries have reported the benefit of short door to balloon time to be limited to patients with early presentation.[10-12]

In an attempt to resolve these conflicts about the onset to balloon time and door to balloon time, we evaluated the relation between the two times and the long term clinical outcome of patients with STEMI in a large observational database of patients with acute myocardial infarction in Japan.

Methods

Study population

The Coronary REvascularization Demonstrating Outcome Study in Kyoto (CREDO-Kyoto) acute myocardial infarction registry is a physician initiated, non-company sponsored, multicentre registry that enrolled consecutive patients with acute myocardial infarction having coronary revascularisation within seven days of the onset of symptoms between January 2005 and December 2007 across 26 tertiary hospitals in Japan (supplementary appendix A). The relevant review boards or ethics committees in all 26 participating centres approved the study protocol. Obtaining written informed consent from the patients was unnecessary because of the retrospective nature of the study; however, we excluded those patients who refused participation in the study when contacted at follow-up.

Among 5429 patients enrolled in the CREDO-Kyoto acute myocardial infarction registry, 4444 patients had an admission diagnosis of STEMI and had primary percutaneous coronary intervention, excluding 195 patients who had coronary artery bypass grafting surgery and 790 patients with non-STEMI. The population for this study consisted of the 3391 patients with STEMI who had primary percutaneous coronary intervention within 24 hours of onset and for whom data on onset to balloon time were available (fig 1⇓).

Independent experienced clinical research coordinators from the study management centre collected demographic, angiographic, and procedural data from hospital charts or hospital databases according to pre-specified definitions. They obtained follow-up data from hospital charts or by contacting patients or referring physicians. The median length of follow-up was 1049 (interquartile range 752-1324) days. Complete one year follow-up information was available for 3240 (95.5%) of the 3391 study patients.

Definitions and endpoints

We defined onset to balloon time as the time from onset of symptoms to first balloon inflation during percutaneous coronary intervention. We defined door to balloon time as the time from arrival at the hospital to first balloon inflation during percutaneous coronary intervention, and presentation time denoted the time from symptom onset to arrival at the hospital (fig 2⇓).

The principal outcome measure for this analysis was a composite of death and congestive heart failure. We defined congestive heart failure as admission to hospital for worsening heart failure requiring intravenous drug treatment. We assessed clinical outcomes both at 30 days and up to three years after the onset of STEMI according to onset to balloon time and door to balloon time.

We divided the patients into two groups according to their onset to balloon time to assess the effect of a short onset to balloon time on clinical outcomes. We selected a cut-off point of three hours for short onset to balloon time in light of previously reported data and the distribution of onset to balloon time in this cohort (fig 3⇓, left panel).[13 14] We assessed the effect of short onset to balloon time (≤3 hours) on clinical outcomes in the entire cohort. We also assessed clinical outcomes according to four categories of onset to balloon time (≤3 hours, 3-6 hours, 6-12 hours, and 12-24 hours). As a subgroup analysis, we compared the effects of short onset to balloon time on the incidences of a composite of death and congestive heart failure among the subgroups with or without risk factors such as heart failure, advanced age, anterior myocardial infarction, renal insufficiency, and multivessel disease.

We also divided the patients into two groups according door to balloon time. We set the cut-off point of 90 minutes for short door to balloon time according to the recommendation in the ACC/AHA guideline for STEMI.[3] We assessed the effect of short door to balloon time (≤90 minutes) on the principal outcome measure in the entire cohort and in the subgroups of patients with early presentation (≤2 hours after symptom onset) and delayed presentation (>2 hours after symptom onset). We selected the cut-off point of two hours for early presentation in light of previously reported data and the distribution of the presentation time in this cohort (fig 3⇓, right panel).[5 10 11]

3編　受動態より能動態を使う／％は分子分母も併記する

Statistical analysis

We present continuous variables as the mean and standard deviation or median and interquartile range and categorical variables as numbers and percentages. We compared categorical variables with the χ² test when appropriate; otherwise, we used Fisher's exact test. We compared continuous variables with Student's t test or a Wilcoxon rank-sum test on the basis of the distribution. We used the Kaplan-Meier method to estimate cumulative incidences of clinical event rates and assessed differences with the log-rank test.

We used a multivariable Cox proportional hazards model stratified by centres to estimate the hazard ratio of short onset to balloon time for a composite of death and congestive heart failure by adjusting for 41 clinically relevant variables (listed in supplementary table A). We dichotomised the continuous variables such as age or body mass index by clinical reference values or median values. We developed Cox proportional hazard models incorporating the same risk adjusting variables to estimate the effect of short door to balloon time in patients with early presentation (≤2 hours after symptom onset) and in those with delayed presentation (>2 hours after symptom onset). We added an interaction variable between the time to presentation (early versus delayed) and door to balloon time (short versus long) in the model of the entire study population to assess whether the effect size of a door to balloon time of 90 minutes or less relative to more than 90 minutes differed between the two groups of patients with early and delayed presentations.

A physician (HS) and a statistician (TM) used JMP 7 and SAS 9.2 to do all the analyses. All the reported P values are two sided. We regarded a P value under 0.05 as statistically significant.

Results

Presentation, baseline characteristics, and drugs according to onset to balloon time

The median onset to balloon time in the entire study population was 4.2 (interquartile range 2.9-7.3) hours. The median times in the short and the delayed onset to balloon time groups were 2.4 (2.0-2.7) hours and 5.5 (4.0-9.4) hours. The rate of achievement of a door to balloon time of 90 minutes or less was significantly higher in the short onset to balloon time group than in the delayed onset to balloon time group (table⇓).

Baseline characteristics differed significantly in several aspects between the short and delayed onset to balloon time groups (table⇓). Patients with advanced age, previous stroke, and anaemia were more common in the delayed onset to balloon time group, whereas the short onset to balloon time group included more patients who were current smokers and had unstable haemodynamics such as cardiogenic shock (Killip class 4) at presentation. The delayed onset to balloon time group included more patients with multivessel disease and a culprit lesion of left circumflex artery, whereas a culprit lesion of left main coronary artery was more prevalent in the short onset to balloon time group (table⇓). The use of statins and β blockers at discharge from hospital was significantly more prevalent in the short onset to balloon time group (table⇓).

Clinical outcomes: short versus delayed onset to balloon time

The three year incidence of a composite of death and congestive heart failure in patients with short onset to balloon time was significantly lower than that in patients with delayed onset to balloon time (13.5% (123 events/964 patients) v 19.2% (429/2427), P<0.001; relative risk reduction 29.7%) (fig 4⇓, top left). An incremental increase in the three year incidence of a composite of death and congestive heart failure was apparent as the onset to balloon time increased from three hours or less to 12-24 hours (fig 4⇓, top right). After adjustment for confounders, an onset to balloon time of three hours or less remained associated with a lower risk of a composite of death and congestive heart failure (adjusted hazard ratio 0.70, 95% confidence interval 0.56 to 0.88; P=0.002). The three year incidence of all cause death in patients with short onset to balloon time was also significantly lower than that in patients with delayed onset to balloon time (10.4% (94/964) v 14.6% (323/2427), P=0.009; relative risk reduction 28.8%) (fig 4⇓, bottom left) and tended to be lower than those in the remaining three categories with delayed onset to balloon time (fig 4⇓, bottom right).

In the subgroup analysis according to the risk profile of the patients, the trend for better clinical outcome in patients with short onset to balloon time was consistent regardless of the presence or absence of risk factors such as heart failure, advanced age, anterior myocardial infarction, renal insufficiency, and multivessel disease, although the absolute differences in the incidences of events were greater in patients at high risk (fig 5⇓ and fog 6⇓).

Presentation, baseline characteristics, and drugs according to door to balloon time

The median door to balloon time in the entire study population was 90 (60-132) minutes. The median time in the short and long door to balloon time groups were 60 (48-78) minutes and 132 (108-168) minutes. The onset to balloon time was significantly shorter in the short than in the long door to balloon time group—3.7 (2.5-6.5) hours versus 4.7 (3.3-7.8) hours (P<0.001).

Patients with advanced age, body mass index below 25, diabetes treated with insulin, heart failure, lower ejection fraction, severe mitral regurgitation, and previous myocardial infarction were more common in the long door to balloon time group, whereas the short door to balloon time group included more current smokers. The long door to balloon time group included more patients with multivessel disease and a culprit lesion of left circumflex artery, whereas a culprit lesion of left main coronary artery or proximal left descending artery was more prevalent in the short door to balloon time group. The use of statins and nitrates at hospital discharge was significantly more prevalent in the short door to balloon time group, whereas cilostazol and nicorandil were more often used in the long door to balloon time group (supplementary table B).

Clinical outcomes: short versus long door to balloon time

In the entire study population, we found no significant difference in the incidence of a composite of death and congestive heart failure (16.7% (270/1671) v 18.4% (282/1720), P=0.54; relative risk reduction 9.2%) or all cause death (12.4% (198/1671) v 14.4% (219/1720), P=0.21; 13.9%) between the two groups of patients with short and long door to balloon time (fig 7⇓, top). However, when we stratified patients by presentation time, short as compared with long door to balloon time was associated with significantly lower incidence of a composite of death and congestive heart failure in patients presenting early (≤2 hours after symptom onset) (11.9% (74/883) v 18.1% (147/655), P=0.01; relative risk reduction 34.3%), but not those presenting later (>2 hours after symptom onset) (19.7% (196/788) v 18.7% (135/1065), P=0.44; −5.3%) (fig 7⇓, bottom). After adjusting for confounders, we found no significant difference in the risk of a composite of death and congestive heart failure between the two groups of patients with short and long door to balloon time (adjusted hazard ratio 0.98, 0.78 to 1.24; P=0.87). Short door to balloon time was independently associated with a lower risk of a composite of death and congestive heart failure in patients with early presentation (adjusted hazard ratio 0.58, 0.38 to 0.87; P=0.009) but not in those with delayed presentation (1.57, 1.12 to 2.18; P=0.008). A significant interaction existed between door to balloon time (≤90 or >90 minutes) and the time to presentation (≤2 or >2 hours after symptom onset) (interaction P=0.01).

Short term versus long term clinical outcomes

Although the long term (three year) incidences of the principal outcome measure and all cause mortality were significantly lower in patients with short onset to balloon time, the short term (30 day) outcome did not differ between the short and delayed onset to balloon time groups in terms of all cause mortality (5.0% (48/964) v 5.2% (125/2427), P=0.82) and a composite of death and congestive heart failure (5.2% (50/964) v 5.5% (133/2427), P=0.71). A trend towards better clinical outcome with short door to balloon time in patients with early presentation was already apparent at 30 days both for all cause death (4.3% (28/883) v 5.7% (50/655), P=0.23) and for a composite of death and congestive heart failure (4.3% (28/883) v 5.9% (52/655), P=0.16) (fig 8⇓).

Discussion

The main findings of this analysis are that a short onset to balloon time of less than three hours was associated with a lower risk of a composite of death and congestive heart failure up to three years of follow-up in patients with ST segment elevation myocardial infarction having primary percutaneous coronary intervention but that the benefit of a short door to balloon time of less than 90 minutes for clinical outcome was limited to patients who presented early.

Comparison with other studies

The large US national registry of myocardial infarction (NRMI) reported that short door to balloon time but not short onset to balloon time was associated with lower in-hospital mortality.[6 7] However, consistent with the results from several smaller studies, our analysis showed a clear association between a short onset to balloon time of less than three hours and better long term clinical outcome. Theoretically, short onset to balloon time, meaning short total ischaemic time, would be expected to be associated with better clinical outcome, because experimental studies have suggested that the effect of reperfusion on myocardial salvage is markedly decreased within two or three hours after the onset of myocardial infarction.[13 15] In actual clinical practice, the correlation between short onset to balloon time and decreased mortality could be unclear because of the uncertainty about symptom onset, survivor bias, variations in the time course of development of myocardial necrosis, and very low in-hospital mortality in the era of primary percutaneous coronary intervention. One of the possible reasons for the discrepancy in the relation of onset to balloon time to clinical outcome between the NRMI study and our study might be a difference in the timeframe of endpoint evaluation—in-hospital event in the NRMI registry and three year event in this study. Clinical outcome at 30 days did not differ between the short and delayed onset to balloon time groups in our study. In-hospital mortality could be affected more by clinical conditions at presentation than by small differences in onset to balloon time or door to balloon time.

Implications of study

Guidelines emphasise the target of a door to balloon time of 90 minutes or less, and the rate at which this is achieved has improved in recent years.[1 16 17] The emphasis on the importance of short door to balloon time was mainly derived from the result of the NRMI, which suggested that short door to balloon time was associated with lower in-hospital mortality regardless of time from symptom onset to presentation. However, our study, in line with several previous studies, suggests that better in-hospital and long term outcome in patients with short door to balloon time was seen only in those patients who presented early.[10 11] The door to balloon time is a part of the onset to balloon time, and, theoretically, the relative importance of door to balloon time would decrease with increasing onset to balloon time. Flynn et al reported that an observed reduction in the door to balloon time between 2003 and 2008 did not lead to significant reduction in in-hospital mortality rates, suggesting that successful implementation of efforts to reduce door to balloon time has not resulted in the expected survival benefits.[18]

Therefore, we should focus more on reducing the onset to balloon time rather than focusing too much on the door to balloon time, although we should continue to make efforts to reduce the door to balloon time in patients presenting early. Further improvement in the outcome of patients with STEMI could be achieved by reducing the total ischaemic time with efforts such as social activities to raise awareness for patients to attend hospital early and improvement of pre-hospital care systems. Finally, all healthcare professionals, including primary care doctors, paramedics, acute physicians, and emergency department staff, as well as cardiologists, should make every effort to promote widespread awareness of the importance of shortening the onset to balloon time in saving the lives of patients with STEMI.

Limitations of study

This study has several limitations. Firstly, we could not exclude the influences of patients' recall bias for symptom onset. Therefore, we accept that exactly the same difficulty found in other studies regarding symptom onset applies to our own study and might partly account not only for the discordance of our findings compared with other studies but also for the internal discordance of late versus early benefit of short onset to balloon time. Secondly, clinical outcomes could have been affected by survivor bias and by variations in the time course of development of myocardial necrosis. Thirdly, risk adjustment by using dichotomised variables had the potential for residual confounding. In addition, treating some variables as continuous variables theoretically improves the power to detect differences.[19] However, we consistently dichotomised the continuous variables in our reports based on the current registry because those dichotomised variables are more easily understood by general physicians. Finally, the huge differences in baseline characteristics between patients with early reperfusion and those with delayed reperfusion might limit the comparability of the groups, although we intended to adjust as extensively as possible to minimise the influence of unmeasured confounders.

Conclusions

Short onset to balloon time was associated with better three year clinical outcome in patients with STEMI having primary percutaneous coronary intervention, whereas the benefit of short

3編　受動態より能動態を使う／％は分子分母も併記する

door to balloon time was limited to patients with early presentation. Efforts to minimise onset to balloon time, including reduction in patient related delays, should be recommended to improve clinical outcome of STEMI patients.

We thank the members of the cardiac catheterisation laboratories of the participating centres and the clinical research coordinators.

Contributors: TK, YN, YF, AN, SS, RT, KY, KN, TS, HM, MA, HT, TM, HE, and SS developed the study design. HS, YN, TM, and TK did the data analysis and drafted the manuscript. TK obtained funding and supervised the study. All authors contributed to the interpretation of the data and revision of the manuscript. TK is the guarantor.

Funding: This study was supported by the Pharmaceuticals and Medical Devices Agency (PMDA) in Japan. The PMDA had no role in the study design; in the collection, analysis, and interpretation of data; in the writing of the reports; or in the decision to submit the article for publication.

Competing interests: All authors have completed the Unified Competing Interest form at www.icmje.org/coi_disclosure.pdf (available on request from the corresponding author) and declare: no support from any organisation for the submitted work; no financial relationships with any organisations that might have an interest in the submitted work in the previous three years; no other relationships or activities that could appear to have influenced the submitted work.

Ethical approval: The protocol for the study was approved by the human research ethics committees of the Kyoto University Graduate School of Medicine.

Data sharing: No additional data available.

1. Gibson C, Pride Y, Frederick P, Pollackjr C, Canto J, Tiefenbrunn A, et al. Trends in reperfusion strategies, door-to-needle and door-to-balloon times, and in-hospital mortality among patients with ST-segment elevation myocardial infarction enrolled in the national registry of myocardial infarction from 1990 to 2006. Am Heart J 2008;156:1035-44.
2. Eagle KA, Nallamothu BK, Mehta RH, Granger CB, Steg PG, Van de Werf F, et al. Trends in acute reperfusion therapy for ST-segment elevation myocardial infarction from 1999 to 2006: we are getting better but we have got a long way to go. Eur Heart J 2008;29:609-17.
3. Antman EM, Anbe DT, Armstrong PW, Bates ER, Green LA, Hand M, et al. ACC/AHA guidelines for the management of patients with ST-elevation myocardial infarction: a report of the American College of Cardiology/American Heart Association Task Force on Practice Guidelines (Committee to Revise the 1999 Guidelines for the Management of Patients with Acute Myocardial Infarction). Circulation 2004;110:e82-292.
4. Antman EM, Hand M, Armstrong PW, Bates ER, Green LA, Halasyamani LK, et al. 2007 focused update of the ACC/AHA 2004 guidelines for the management of patients with ST-elevation myocardial infarction: a report of the American College of Cardiology/American Heart Association Task Force on Practice Guidelines: developed in collaboration with the Canadian Cardiovascular Society endorsed by the American Academy of Family Physicians. Circulation 2007;117:296-329.
5. Van de Werf F, Bax J, Betriu A, Blomstrom-Lundqvist C, Crea F, Falk V, et al. Management of acute myocardial infarction in patients presenting with persistent ST-segment elevation: the task force on the management of ST-segment elevation acute myocardial infarction of the European Society of Cardiology. Eur Heart J 2008;29:2909-45.
6. Cannon CP. Relationship of symptom-onset-to-balloon time and door-to-balloon time with mortality in patients undergoing angioplasty for acute myocardial infarction. JAMA 2000;283:2941-7.
7. McNamara R, Wang Y, Herrin J, Curtis J, Bradley E, Magid D, et al. Effect of door-to-balloon time on mortality in patients with ST segment elevation myocardial infarction. J Am Coll Cardiol 2006;47:2180-6.
8. De Luca G, Suryapranata H, Zijlstra F, van't Hof AWJ, Hoorntje JCA, Gosselink ATM, et al. Symptom-onset-to-balloon time and mortality in patients with acute myocardial infarction treated by primary angioplasty. J Am Coll Cardiol 2003;42:991-7.
9. Brodie BR, Stuckey TD, Wall TC, Kissling G, Hansen CJ, Muncy DB, et al. Importance of time to reperfusion for 30-day and late survival and recovery of left ventricular function after primary angioplasty for acute myocardial infarction. J Am Coll Cardiol 1998;32:1312-9.
10. Brodie B, Hansen C, Stuckey T, Richter S, Versteeg D, Gupta N, et al. Door-to-balloon time with primary percutaneous coronary intervention for acute myocardial infarction impacts late cardiac mortality in high-risk patients and patients presenting early after the onset of symptoms. J Am Coll Cardiol 2006;47:289-95.
11. Brodie BR, Gersh BJ, Stuckey T, Witzenbichler B, Guagliumi G, Peruga JZ, et al. When is door-to-balloon time critical? Analysis from the HORIZONS-AMI (Harmonizing Outcomes with Revascularization and Stents in Acute Myocardial Infarction) and CADILLAC (Controlled Abciximab and Device Investigation to Lower Late Angioplasty Complications) trials. J Am Coll Cardiol 2010;56:407-13.
12. Hannan EL, Zhong Y, Jacobs AK, Holmes DR, Walford G, Venditti FJ, et al. Effect of onset-to-door time and door-to-balloon time on mortality in patients undergoing percutaneous coronary interventions for ST-segment elevation myocardial infarction. Am J Cardiol 2010;106:143-7.
13. Gersh BJ. Pharmacological facilitation of primary percutaneous coronary intervention for acute myocardial infarction: is the slope of the curve the shape of the future? JAMA 2005;293:979-86.
14. Boden W, Eagle K, Granger C. Reperfusion strategies in acute ST-segment elevation myocardial infarction: a comprehensive review of contemporary management options. J Am Coll Cardiol 2007;50:917-29.
15. Gersh BJ, Anderson JL. Thrombolysis and myocardial salvage: results of clinical trials and the animal paradigm—paradoxic or predictable? Circulation 1993;88:296-306.
16. Krumholz H. A campaign to improve the timeliness of primary percutaneous coronary intervention door-to-balloon: an alliance for quality. JACC Cardiovasc Interv 2008;1:97-104.
17. Bradley EH, Nallamothu BK, Herrin J, Ting HH, Stern AF, Nembhard IM, et al. National efforts to improve door-to-balloon time results from the door-to-balloon alliance. J Am Coll Cardiol 2009;54:2423-9.
18. Flynn A, Moscucci M, Share D, Smith D, LaLonde T, Changezi H, et al. Trends in door-to-balloon time and mortality in patients with ST-elevation myocardial infarction undergoing primary percutaneous coronary intervention. Arch Intern Med 2010;170:1842-9.
19. Altman DG, Royston P. The cost of dichotomising continuous variables. BMJ 2006;332:1080.

Accepted: 05 April 2012

Cite this as: BMJ 2012;344:e3257

This is an open-access article distributed under the terms of the Creative Commons Attribution Non-commercial License, which permits use, distribution, and reproduction in any medium, provided the original work is properly cited, the use is non commercial and is otherwise in compliance with the license. See: http://creativecommons.org/licenses/by-nc/2.0/ and http://creativecommons.org/licenses/by-nc/2.0/legalcode.

What is already known on this topic

- Results from previous studies are quite inconsistent regarding the relation of symptom onset to balloon time and clinical outcomes in patients with ST segment elevation myocardial infarction
- The time to evaluate endpoints varied widely between these different studies
- Little is known about the relation of onset to balloon time with long term clinical outcomes in actual clinical practice

What this study adds

- A clear association has been shown between a short onset to balloon time of less than three hours and better long term (three year) clinical outcomes
- The benefit of short door to balloon time was limited to patients who presented early
- Further improvement in the outcome of patients with ST segment elevation myocardial infarction could be achieved by reducing the total ischaemic time with various efforts

Table

Table 1 | Patients' characteristics. Values are numbers (percentages) unless stated otherwise

	Entire cohort (n=3391)	Onset to balloon time ≤3 hours (n=964)	Onset to balloon time >3 hours (n=2427)	P value
Baseline characteristics				
Mean (SD) age (years)	67.5 (12.2)	65.3 (12.0)	68.3 (12.2)	<0.001
Male sex	2512 (74)	768 (80)	1744 (72)	<0.001
Mean (SD) body mass index (kg/m^2)	23.5 (3.4)	23.8 (3.4)	23.5 (3.4)	0.01
Hypertension	2660 (78)	741 (77)	1919 (79)	0.16
Diabetes mellitus	1066 (31)	311 (32)	755 (31)	0.51
Treated with insulin	145 (4.3)	41 (4.3)	104 (4.3)	0.97
Current smoker	1380 (41)	445 (46)	935 (39)	<0.001
Heart failure	1050 (31)	304 (32)	746 (31)	0.65
Mean (SD) ejection fraction	52.6 (12.6)	53.6 (12.7)	52.1 (12.6)	0.005
Previous myocardial infarction	293 (8.6)	101 (10)	192 (7.9)	0.02
Previous stroke (with symptoms)	288 (8.5)	64 (6.6)	224 (9.2)	0.01
Peripheral vascular disease	102 (3.0)	25 (2.6)	77 (3.2)	0.37
Median (IQR) eGFR (mL/min/1.73m^2)*	69.4 (54.2-85.4)	68.0 (53.4-82.0)	70.3 (54.5-86.5)	0.03
Atrial fibrillation	314 (9.3)	98 (10)	216 (8.9)	0.26
Anaemia (haemoglobin <11.0 g/dL)	309 (9.1)	63 (6.5)	246 (10)	<0.001
Chronic obstructive pulmonary disease	106 (3.1)	27 (2.8)	79 (3.3)	0.49
Presentation				
Median (IQR) hours from onset to presentation	2.4 (1.1-5.1)	0.9 (0.6-1.3)	3.4 (2.0-7.0)	<0.001
Median (IQR) hours from onset to balloon	4.2 (2.9-7.3)	2.4 (2.0-2.7)	5.5 (4.0-9.4)	<0.001
Hours from onset to balloon:				
<3	964 (28)	964 (100)	0 (0)	<0.001
3-6	1359 (40)	0 (0)	1359 (56)	
6-12	659 (19)	0 (0)	659 (27)	
12-24	409 (12)	0 (0)	409 (17)	
Median (IQR) minutes from door to balloon	90 (60-132)	78 (54-102)	102 (66-150)	<0.001
≤90 minutes from door to balloon	1720 (51)	635 (66)	1085 (45)	<0.001
Haemodynamics:				
Killip class 1	2551 (75)	700 (73)	1851 (76)	<0.001
Killip class 2	283 (8.3)	65 (6.7)	218 (9.0)	
Killip class 3	85 (2.5)	17 (1.8)	68 (2.8)	
Killip class 4	472 (14)	182 (19)	290 (12)	
Intra-aortic balloon pump use	528 (16)	172 (18)	356 (15)	0.02

3編　受動態より能動態を使う／%は分子分母も併記する

Table 1 (continued)

	Entire cohort (n=3391)	Onset to balloon time ≤3 hours (n=964)	Onset to balloon time >3 hours (n=2427)	P value
Angiographic characteristics				
Infarct related artery location:				
Left anterior descending artery	1577 (47)	432 (45)	1145 (47)	<0.001
Left circumflex artery	331 (9.8)	72 (7.5)	259 (11)	
Right coronary artery	1395 (41)	424 (44)	971 (40)	
Left main coronary artery	73 (2.2)	32 (3.3)	41 (1.7)	
Coronary artery bypass graft	15 (0.4)	4 (0.4)	11 (0.5)	
Multivessel disease	1714 (51)	455 (47)	1259 (52)	0.01
Drugs at discharge				
Thienopyridine	3257 (96)	926 (96)	2331 (96)	0.99
Aspirin	3348 (99)	950 (99)	2398 (99)	0.55
Statins	1823 (54)	549 (57)	1274 (52)	0.02
β blockers	1381 (41)	419 (43)	962 (40)	0.04
ACE inhibitor/ARB	2447 (72)	705 (73)	1742 (72)	0.43
Nitrates	1020 (30)	294 (31)	726 (30)	0.74
Calcium channel blockers	649 (19)	189 (20)	460 (19)	0.66

ACE=angiotensin converting enzyme; ARB=angiotensin receptor blocker; IQR=interquartile range.
*Estimated glomerular filtration rate calculated by modification of diet in renal disease formula modified for Japanese patients.

Figures

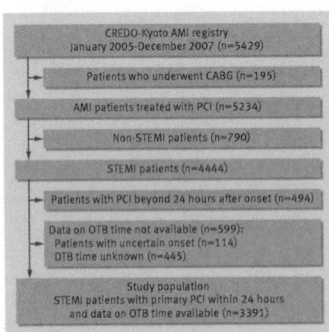

Fig 1 Flow chart for selection of study population. AMI=acute myocardial infarction; DTB=door to balloon time; OTB=onset to balloon; PCI=percutaneous coronary intervention; STEMI=ST segment elevation myocardial infarction

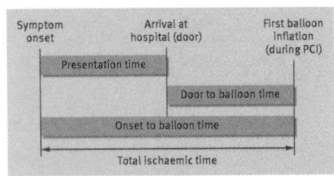

Fig 2 Schema for timeframe from symptom onset to primary percutaneous coronary intervention (PCI)

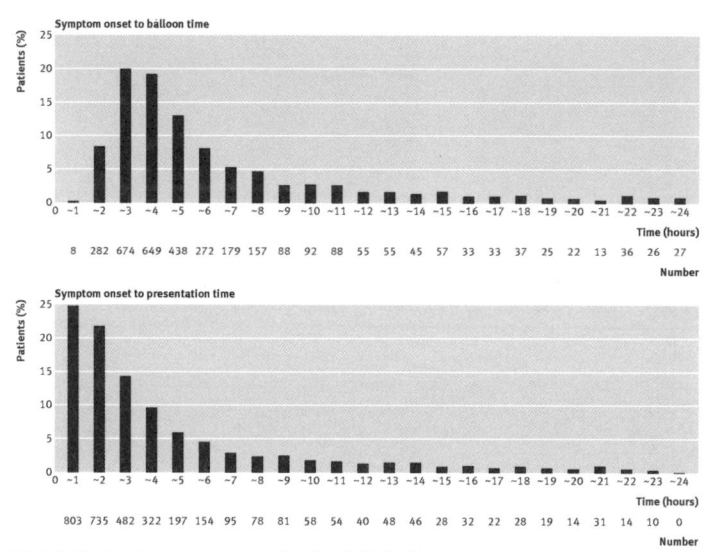

Fig 3 Distribution of symptom onset to balloon time (left); distribution of symptom onset to hospital presentation time (right)

3編　受動態より能動態を使う／％は分子分母も併記する

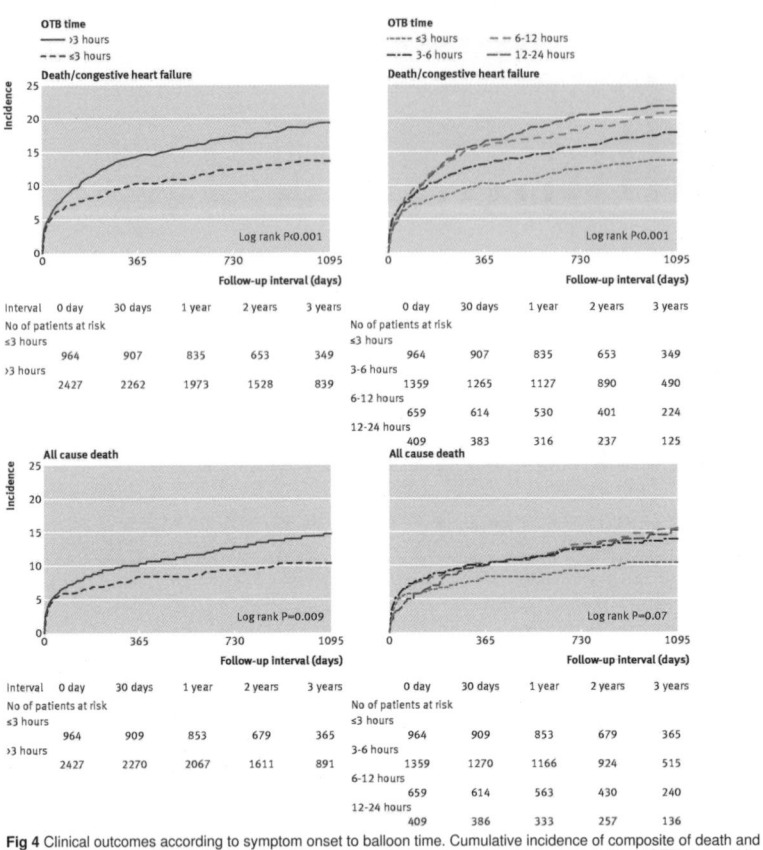

Fig 4 Clinical outcomes according to symptom onset to balloon time. Cumulative incidence of composite of death and congestive heart failure (CHF) was compared between two groups of patients with onset to balloon (OTB) time within and over three hours (top left) and among four OTB time categories (top right). Cumulative incidences of all cause death were also compared between two groups of patients with OTB time within and over three hours (bottom left) and among four OTB time categories (bottom right)

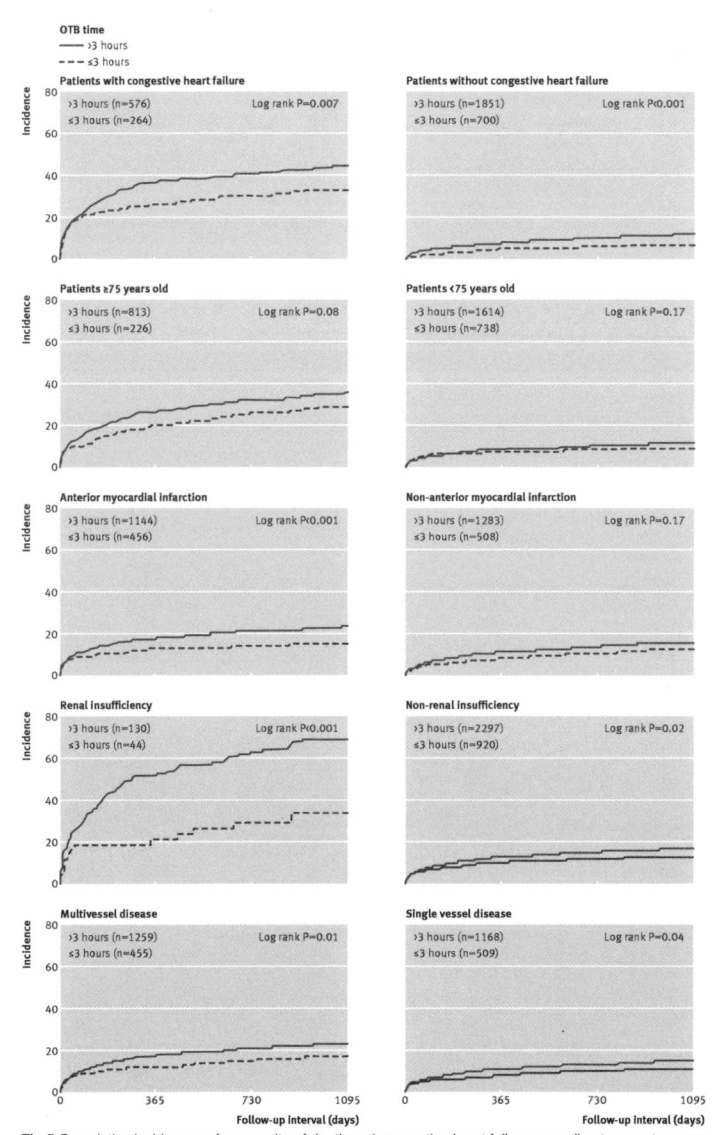

Fig 5 Cumulative incidences of composite of death and congestive heart failure according to symptom onset to balloon (OTB) time stratified by risk profile of patients

3編　受動態より能動態を使う／％は分子分母も併記する

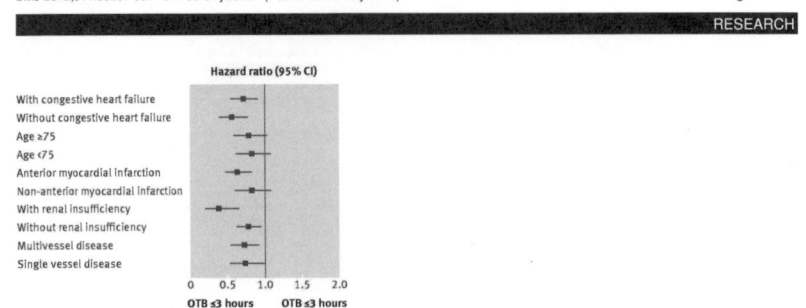

Fig 6 Hazard ratios of short versus delayed symptom onset to balloon (OTB) time for composite of death and congestive heart failure stratified by risk profile of patients

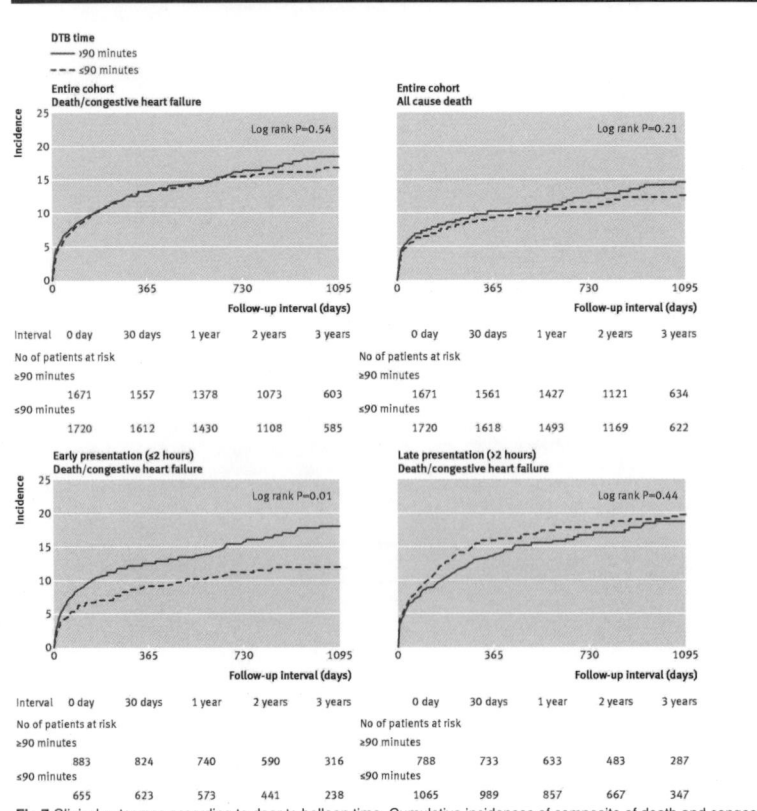

Fig 7 Clinical outcomes according to door to balloon time. Cumulative incidences of composite of death and congestive heart failure (CHF) (top left) and all cause death (top right) were compared between two groups of patients with door to balloon (DTB) time within and over 90 minutes in entire cohort. Cumulative incidences of composite of death and CHF were also compared between two groups of patients with DTB time within and over 90 minutes in patients with early presentation (≤2 hours after symptom onset) (bottom left) and in those with delayed presentation (>2 hours after symptom onset) (bottom right)

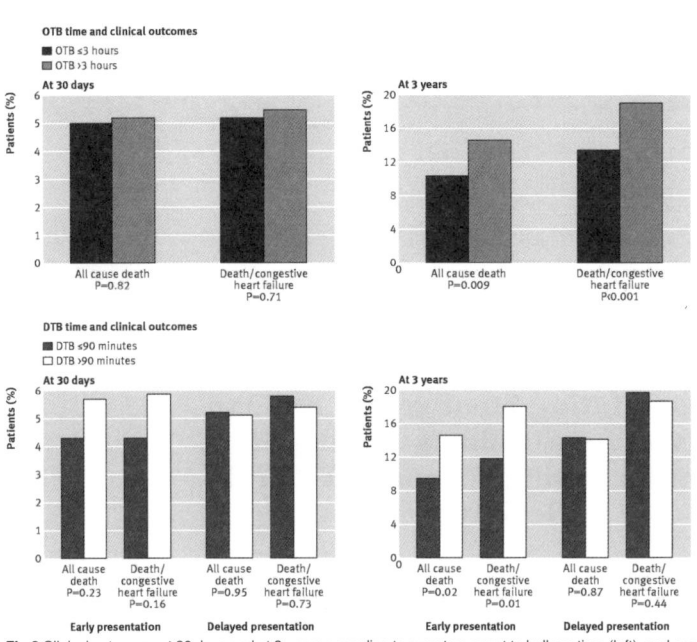

Fig 8 Clinical outcomes at 30 days and at 3 years according to symptom onset to balloon time (left), and according to door to balloon time (right)

(Shiomi H, et al.：Association of onset to balloon and door to balloon time with long term clinical outcome in patients with ST elevation acute myocardial infarction having primary percutaneous coronary intervention: observational study. *BMJ* 2012;344:e3257. 許諾を得て転載)

4編 表現は明確に 結論は結果から導き出される主たるメッセージ

Before

Sirolimus-Eluting Stent versus Balloon Angioplasty for Sirolimus-Eluting Stent Restenosis: Insights from j-CYPHER Registry

Mitsuru Abe, MD; Takuya Taniguchi, MD;
Takeshi Morimoto, MD, MPH;
Futoshi Yamanaka, MD; Kazuhiro Nakao, MD;
Nobuhito Yagi, MD; Nobuaki Kokubu, MD;
Yoichiro Kasahara, MD; Yu Kataoka, MD;
Yoritaka Otsuka, MD; Atsushi Kawamura, MD;
Kazuaki Mitsudo, MD; Takeshi Kimura, MD;
Hiroshi Nonogi, MD; For the j-CYPHER Registry Investigators

From the Division of Cardiology (M.A., T.T., F.Y., K.N., N.Y., N.K., Y.Kasahara, Y.Kataoka, Y.O., H.N.), National Cardiovascular Center, Suita, Japan; Division of Internal Medicine (A.K.), Certral Hospital, Fukuyama, Japan; Center for Medical Education (T.M.) and Department of Cardiovascular Medicine (T.K.), Graduate School of Medicine, Kyoto University, Kyoto, Japan; Division of Cardiology (M.K.), Kurashiki Central Hospital, Kurashiki, Japan.

A Short Title: SES vs. BA for SES restenosis
MANUSCRIPT ID:
The Total Word Count: 5507 words

Correspondence to Takeshi Kimura, Department of Cardiovascular Medicine, Graduate School of Medicine, Kyoto University, 54 Shogoin, Kawahara-cho, Sakyo-ku, Kyoto, 606-8507, Japan
Fax number: xxxx
Telephone number: xxxx
E-mail address: xxxx

Abstract

Background
The widespread use of sirolimus-eluting stents (SES) to complex lesions is associated with higher rate of target lesion revascularization (TLR) in real-world clinical practice. There is, however, limited information about optimal treatment of SES restenosis.

Methods and Results
In the j-CYPHER registry, we identified ① **1055 patients with 1164 lesions** of SES restenosis treated with SES (551 lesions) or balloon angioplasty (BA) (613 lesions) at their operators' discretion. ＊ ② The incidences of second TLR within 1-year and 2-year were 17.0% and 23.7% in lesions implanted with SES and 32.0% and 37.1% in lesions treated with BA, respectively. ③ Among them, one year follow-up was completed with 412 lesions in 383 SES-treated patients and 454 lesions in 426 BA-treated patients. We identified 8 univariate correlates of second TLR within 1 year after SES implantation. After adjustment for these factors, SES implantation (vs. BA) was revealed to have a significantly lower rate of 2nd TLR after treatment of SES restenosis (OR, 0.45; 95%CI, 0.33 to 0.63; $P<0.001$). The ④ overall mortality ($P=0.1$) and cumulative rates of stent thrombosis ($P=0.7$) were ⑤ not significantly different between two groups.

Conclusions
Repeat SES implantation is more effective than and is as safe as BA for the treatment of SES restenosis in our study population.

Keywords
restenosis, angioplasty, stents, balloon

Abstractの限られた字数の中で, 総論的なIntroductionは不要.

①1055人, 1164病変になるまでの母集団の情報がほしい.

＊結果を書く前に何をエンドポイントとしてみたいのかを記載.

②4つの数字があるが, 1年と2年を比べたいのか, SESとBAを比べたいのか明確にし, 2つの数字の比較にしたほうがわかりやすい.

③次の多変量解析の前段階でありAbstractでは省略してよい.

④時間枠を記載.

⑤具体的な数字を記載し, そこにP値を移す.

Sirolimus-eluting stents (SES) significantly reduce the rate of angiographic restenosis and target lesion revascularization (TLR), but the widespread use of SES to complex lesions is associated with higher rate of TLR in real-world clinical practice.

In patients with bare-metal stent restenosis, several prospective, multicenter, randomized trials demonstrated that the implantation of SES was superior to balloon angioplasty (BA), implantation of bare-metal stent, or vascular brachytherapy. Although a few previous studies reported that the use of SES was associated with a lower TLR rate compared with BA., there is limited information about comparison of SES implantation with BA for the treatment of SES restenosis.

As for concerns of a potentially higher risk of death or stent thrombosis associated with repeat SES implantation to SES restenosis, we also evaluated the incidences of those events after treatment with SES or BA.

> 直前まで再狭窄の再治療の話だったのに、ここだけは突然初回の治療の話に読めるので、recurrent の TLR であることを明確に。
>
> a few previous studies と limited information は同じこと。何が言いたいのか明確に。

Methods

Patients

The j-CYPHER registry is a physician-initiated prospective, multi-center observational study in Japan enrolling consecutive patients undergoing SES implantation, and the study protocol and main results were reported elsewhere. The relevant review boards in all 37 participating centers approved the study protocol. Written informed consent was obtained from all patients.

The inclusion criteria were the enrollment of j-CYPHER registry and TLR for SES restenosis with repeat SES implantation or BA-treatment. The exclusion criteria were treatment for SES restenosis with combination of SES and BA in analysis for mortality after first TLR, and the occurrence of stent thrombosis at first TLR in analysis for stent thrombosis after first TLR.

Definitions

*

Coronary angiographic parameters were assessed in each participating center either by visual assessment or by quantitative angiographic measurement. Lesion complexity was determined by the operator. The other definitions of bifurcation lesion, death, myocardial infarction, and stent thrombosis were described previously.

> ＊プライマリポイントとセカンダリアウトカムをここで明確にする。また、後のリスクファクターの解析で用いられる変数で、特殊なもの（例：ostial lesion）はここで定義しておく。

Age was dichotomized to elderly or not (≥80 years old vs. <80 years old), body mass index dichotomized to obese or not (body mass index ≥25.0 vs. <25.0), ejection fraction dichotomized to poor left ventricle systolic function or not (ejection fraction ≤40% vs. >40%), lesion characteristics dichotomized to complex or not (B2 and C vs. A and B1), lesion length dichotomized to long or not (lesion length ≥30 mm vs. <30 mm), and preprocedural reference diameter dichotomized to small or not (reference diameter <2.5 mm vs. ≥2.5 mm).

For risk factor analysis, TLR was defined as treatment for SES restenosis with repeat SES implantation or BA within 365 days after first TLR. Those without TLR within 365 days was considered no TLR.

Statistical Analysis

Continuous variables were presented with mean ± standard deviation and the categorical variables are expressed as number and percentages. Categorical variables were compared with the chi-square test. Continuous variables were compared with the t test or Wilcoxon rank sum test based on the distribution. Cumulative mortality was estimated by the Kaplan-Meier method, and differences were assessed with the log-rank test.

Based on previous reports demonstrating the association between several factors with TLR after SES implantation, we used the variables included elderly, male gender, obesity, hypertension, diabetes mellitus, current smoking, treatment for hypercholesterolemia, estimated glomerular filtration rate <30 mL/min/1.73m^2 without hemodialysis, hemodialysis, acute coronary syndrome, prior myocardial infarction, prior stroke, peripheral vascular disease, prior heart failure, diseased vessels, poor left ventricle systolic function, emergent procedure, lesion location, de novo lesion, in-stent restenosis, ST-elevation myocardial infarction culprit lesion, ostial location, chronic total occlusion, severe calcification, bifurcation lesion, complex lesion, long lesion, small vessel, use of intravascular ultrasound, direct stenting, and additional dilatation as potential independent factors responsible for second TLR. The univariate relationships between second TLR and these variables were evaluated by chi-square test. The variables that showed significant correlation (*P* values <0.05) with second TLR were then entered into logistic regression model with variable of SES-implantation (vs. BA). The association was shown as odds ratio (OR) with 95% confidence intervals (CIs) and *P* values. Results were considered as significant with a P value of <0.05. We used JMP 8 (SAS Institute Inc, Cary, NC) for all analyses.

*

Results

Study Population

From August 2004 to November 2006, 15155 patients were enrolled in the registry from 29555 consecutive patients. After the exclusion of 2331 patients who were registered repeatedly, 12824 patients with 19675 lesions were enrolled in the registry for the first time (Figure 1). 12812 patients with 17545 lesions were successfully implanted with at least one SES and 17050 lesions were treated exclusively with SES. Among them, 1298 patients with 1456 lesions (8.5%) were re-treated (first TLR). The median follow-up from the enrollment into the registry to the first TLR was 829 days (interquartile range 498 to 1108 days).

We identified 1055 patients with 1164 lesions of SES restenosis treated with SES (551 lesions) or BA (613 lesions) at their operators' discretion. Lesions treated with BA consisted of 526 plain old balloon-treated lesions and 87 cutting balloon-treated lesions. Treatment of the remaining 292 lesions included coronary artery bypass grafting (69 lesions), bare-metal stent (73 lesions), other types of drug-eluting stent (101 lesions), combination of SES and other stent types (8 lesions), rotational atherectomy (1 lesion), aspiration (1 lesion), unidentified (17 lesions), and failed procedure (22 lesions). Since paclitaxel-eluting stent was not approved for clinical use until May 2007 in Japan, only 94 lesions of SES restenosis were treated with paclitaxel-eluting stent. We excluded paclitaxel-eluting stent-treated lesions because of relatively short median follow-up days (225 days, interquartile range 43 to 350 days). Because 25 patients were treated with combination of SES (28 lesions) and BA (30 lesions), 1055 patients with 1164 lesions were consisted of 511 patients with 551 SES-treated lesions and 569 patients with 613 BA-treated lesions. Cumulative mortality was calculated for 486 patients treated with only SES and 544 patients treated with only BA, and compared between treatment. Factors associated with second TLR for all 1164 lesions were evaluated. In total, one year follow-up was completed with 412 lesions treated with SES and 454 lesions treated with BA, and 242 lesions were re-treated within 1 year

*スポンサーのある研究であり、そのスポンサーと深い関連のある治療法の論文なので、スポンサーの役割を記載すること.

and 624 lesions were free from revascularization during 1 year. Because we excluded 70 lesions with stent thrombosis at first TLR, 1094 lesions consisted of 537 lesions treated with SES and 557 lesions treated with BA were analyzed for stent thrombosis after first TLR.

Baseline Patient Characteristics

Baseline patient characteristics were similar between groups except that patients receiving SES have preserved estimated glomerular filtration rate (P=0.02) and ejection fraction (P=0.03), and were more frequent with ST-elevation myocardial infarction (P=0.03). The patients treated with BA were more likely to have diabetes mellitus (P=0.004), especially insulin therapy (P=0.004) (Table 1).

これだけ違うのでsimilarと言うよりはdifferentと言うほうがよい.

Baseline Lesion and Procedural Characteristics

Lesions and procedural characteristics treated with SES were more frequent with saphenous vein graft lesion (P=0.004), de novo lesion (P=0.008), use of intravascular ultrasound (P=0.005), and direct stenting (P=0.0006). Lesions and procedural characteristics treated with BA were more likely to be LCx lesion (P=0.002), in-stent restenosis at index procedure (P<0.0001), side branch stenting (P=0.006), long lesion length (≥30mm) (P=0.03), more stents used (P=0.0004), and longer length stents used (P=0.001) (Table 2).

Mortality

We investigated the incidences of death after first TLR. Among 486 patients treated with only SES and 544 patients treated with only BA, the rates of all-cause mortality within 1-year and 2-year were 4.6% and 10.4% in patients implanted with SES and 7.9% and 12.0% in patients treated with BA, respectively. The overall mortality were not significantly different between two groups (P=0.1) (Figure 1).

この論文の主たる目的が2回目のTLRなので"Mortality"は副次的として後ろにもっていく.

これはsecondary outcomeの解析方法であるので, Methodsのアウトカムへ.

The Incidence and 1-Year rate of Second TLR

Among 551 lesions treated with SES and 613 lesions treated with BA, the incidences of second TLR within 1-year and 2-year were 17.0% and 23.7% in lesions implanted with SES and 32.0% and 37.1% in lesions treated with BA, respectively (Figure 2). Cumulative rate of second TLR after treatment with SES for SES restenosis was significantly lower than that after treatment with BA ($P<0.0001$).

Among 242 lesions re-treated and 624 lesions free from revascularization within 1 year after first TLR, univariate correlates of second TLR were revealed as hemodialysis, prior heart failure, de novo lesion, in-stent restenosis, ST-elevation myocardial infarction culprit lesion at index procedure, severe calcification, use of intravascular ultrasound, and direct stenting (Table 3).

After adjustment for these factors, multivariate logistic regression model showed that repeat SES implantation to SES restenosis compared with treatment with BA was an independent factor for lower rate of second TLR (OR, 0.45; 95%CI, 0.33 to 0.63; $P<0.001$) (Table 4).

*

Incidence of Stent Thrombosis

Among 537 lesions treated with SES and 557 lesions treated with BA, the incidences of definite stent thrombosis within 1-year and 2-year after first TLR were 0.2% and 0.6% in lesions implanted with SES and 0.6% and 0.6% in lesions treated with BA, respectively (Figure 3). Cumulative rates of definite stent thrombosis were not significantly different between two groups ($P=0.7$).

Discussion

We showed that: 1) SES implantation (vs. BA) was revealed to have a significantly lower rate of second TLR within 1 year after treatment for SES restenosis (OR, 0.45; 95%CI, 0.33 to 0.63). 2) repeat SES implantation was not associated with higher mortality comparing to treatment with BA in patients with SES restenosis. 3) Repeat SES implantation did not increase the incidence of stent thrombosis in comparison with BA-treatment.

Baseline patient, lesion, and procedural characteristics were almost similar including age, serum creatinine, the prevalence of hypertension, prior myocardial infarction, prior stroke, prior heart failure, poor left ventricular systolic function, the percentage of male gender, emergent procedure, ostial location, chronic total occlusion, severe calcification, and complex lesion.

The patients and the lesions receiving SES were, however, more associated with preserved estimated glomerular filtration rate and ejection fraction, ST-elevation myocardial infarction,

＊査読の結果，ここに Angiographic Results を入れることになった．

Results の冗長な繰り返しであり，重要性も前のパラグラフほどではない．Discussion が長くなる原因なので削除．

saphenous vein graft lesion, de novo lesion, use of intravascular ultrasound, and direct stenting. The patients and the lesions treated with BA were more likely to have diabetes mellitus and especially insulin therapy, LCx lesion, in-stent restenosis at index procedure, side branch stenting, long lesion length (≥30mm), more stents used, and longer length stents used. Because the strategy of treatment for SES restenosis was at their operators' discretion, this result revealed the tendency and preference of Japanese cardiac interventionists to fix SES restenosis.

Although the results of DELAYED PRISC trial showed that SES implantation was associated with higher mortality than BMS implantation for saphenous vein graft disease, we did not know SES implantation was associated with higher mortality than BA-treatment to SES restenosis in those lesions. But we knew higher rate of TLR in saphenous vein graft lesions, so Japanese physicians had a tendency to implant SES again into SES restenosis in those lesions. The lesions where intravascular ultrasound could be performed had somewhat large lumen profile and were easy to deliver devices, so physicians preferred to repeat SES implantation.

Some previous studies including REALITY trial reported that beneficial effects of SES implantation might be weakened in patients with diabetes, therefore Japanese cardiac interventionists preferred to treat with BA for SES restenosis in patients with diabetes. Because at least two stents were already implanted to the lesion of in-stent restenosis at index procedure, interventionists treated with BA rather than SES implantation again for SES restenosis.

The cumulative incidence of second TLR after repeat SES implantation depicted by the Kaplan-Meier curve was significantly lower compared with that after treatment with BA. The difference occurred and grew larger during first one year and persisted after that. As for bare-metal stent restenosis, the implantation of SES was superior to BA, implantation of bare-metal stent, or vascular brachytherapy. There was, however, limited information regarding whether the implantation of SES is superior to BA-treatment in patients with SES restenosis. Cosgrave et al. identified 250 drug-eluting stent restenosis in 203 patients and divided these lesions into two groups: focal and non-focal. For focal restenotic lesions, the incidence of TLR following drug-eluting stent implantation and BA-treatment was 8.6% and 11.4%, respectively. For non-focal restenotic lesions, that was

22.6% and 24%, respectively. It is interesting to note that Kim et al. reported that the repeated TLR rate at 1 year was 3.3% for the SES group and 8.3% for BA group. The reported incidences of both groups were extremely low compared with other studies including ours. In Kitahara's report, 102 lesions in 101 patients who underwent TLR for SES restenosis were divided into focal or non-focal restenosis. Re-TLR were observed in 12.5% of the focal-drug-eluting stent group, in 35.5% of the focal-BA group, in 35.3% of the non-focal-drug-eluting stent group, and in 50.0% of the non-focal-BA group during the mean follow-up of 13.0 ± 8.9 months. Focal restenosis was associated with lower incidence of target lesion failure compared with non-focal restenosis in case of treatment with bare-metal stent and SES. We did not have enough data about patterns of SES restenosis, but previous reports demonstrated that focal restenosis remained the most common pattern (71.3%-79.0%) with SES in real-world clinical practice.

In our study population, the incidence of target lesion failure following implantation of SES and treatment with BA for SES restenosis within 1 year was 17.0% and 32.0%, respectively. Among 242 lesions re-treated and 624 lesions free from revascularization within 1 year after first TLR, univariate correlates of second TLR were revealed as hemodialysis, prior heart failure, de novo lesion, in-stent restenosis, ST-elevation myocardial infarction culprit lesion at index procedure, severe calcification, use of intravascular ultrasound, and direct stenting. After adjustment for these factors, multivariate logistic regression model showed that repeat SES implantation to SES restenosis compared with treatment with BA was an independent factor for lower rate of second TLR.

ここも Results の繰り返しであり、削ってよい。

As for safety concerns, SES implantation into another SES may lead to several alterations in drug release, hypersensitivity to "double-dose" polymers, and an inadequate stent expansion at the area of stent overlap. One or more of these factors may cause the unexpected events such as death or stent thrombosis. Because of the growing concerns of a potentially higher risk of death and stent thrombosis after drug-eluting stent implantation, we evaluated the incidences of these two events after SES implantation or BA-treatment for SES restenosis. The incidence of all-cause death within 1-year and 2-year after second TLR were 4.6% and 10.4% in patients implanted with SES and 7.9% and 12.0% in patients treated with BA, respectively. The definite stent thrombosis within 1-year and 2-year were observed in 0.2% and

0.6% in lesions with SES and 0.6% and 0.6% in lesions treated with BA, respectively. Although baseline clinical, lesion, and procedural characteristics were not matched between two groups, we could not find any signal that repeat SES implantation may increase the unexpected events such as death or stent thrombosis compared with BA-treatment. Therefore, the implantation of SES was as safe as BA for the treatment of SES restenosis in our study population.

Study limitations

There are several limitations in our study. First, both first and second TLR were follow-up events in the j-CYPHER registry. We had plenty of data on clinical, lesion, and procedural characteristics at index procedure, but we had not planned to obtain enough clinical and angiographic data at the time of TLR. Therefore, we conducted this study based on only baseline characteristics. Second, the outcome, TLR might be depended on their operators' discretion.①Because analysis for TLR was not suitable for survival carve analysis, we used logistic regression model to minimize the bias.② Third, our study included largest population, admitted to 37 centers. However, definite stent thrombosis was a rare event and that we observed was only 2 patients treated with SES and 3 patients treated with BA. The number of patients might not be enough to examine the data of stent thrombosis.③Fourth, the present study was not a randomized trial and all patients underwent second TLR at their operators' discretion. Therefore, some patients were selected to implant SES again because of preexisting clinical, lesion and procedural conditions and others were not. Such situation undoubtedly resulted in selection bias. ＊Fifth, without systematic angiographic follow-up, the obtained TLR may underestimate the 'true' clinical restenosis rate.④Sixth, we can not exclude the potential effect of other unknown confounders.

Conclusions

①The present study enrolled larger number of patients and lesions compared with previous reports, and were conducted in 37 medical centers. Despite limitations,②second TLR occurred in 17.0% of SES-treated lesions and 32.0% of BA-treated lesions during 1 year follow-up after first TLR.③Repeat SES implantation is superior to BA for the treatment of SES restenosis after

---

①これはMethodsで述べる．ほかにTLRが症状が起こって発生したのか，ルーチンの検査で見つかったのかの区別がないことを記載する．

②これは副次的な解析なので外してよい．

③これは本論文の主たる変数についてのlimitationであり，前にもってくる．

＊限界があるだけでなく，結論への影響度について記載する．

④これはコホート研究に必ず発生する問題でlimitationの冒頭に書く．

①これは結果の信頼性を上げるが「結論」ではない．

②これはResultsで述べた．

③これが「結論」．

④ adjustment for risk factors for second TLR. As for death and stent thrombosis, repeat SES implantation was ⑤ as safe as BA for the treatment of SES restenosis in our study population. To validate our results, a large-size randomized and controlled study is needed.

④これは「方法」であり不要.

⑤この部分が結論であり，後は省略可能．

Acknowledgements

The authors are indebted to Hiromi Maeda for secretarial assistance.

Sources of Funding

This study was supported by Cordis Cardiology Japan, a Johnson & Johnson company. The study sponsor was not involved in the study design; in the collection, analysis, and interpretation of data; in the writing of the report; or in the decision to submit the article for publication.

これを Methods に．（しかし，最終的な論文では編集部の判断で削除されている）

Disclosures

Dr Kimura serves as an advisory board member and member of the speakers' bureau for Cordis Cardiology and has received honoraria from Cordis Cardiology. Dr Mitsudo reports receipt of honoraria from Cordis Cardiology. The remaining authors report no conflicts.

References（省略）

Figure Legends

Figure 1
Study population of analysis for mortality, recurrent TLR, and stent thrombosis among patients enrolled for j-CYPHER registry
SES indicates sirolimus-eluting stent; TLR, target lesion revascularization; CABG, coronary artery bypass grafting; BMS, bare-metal stent; DES, drug-eluting stent; and BA, balloon angioplasty.

Figure 2
Cumulative incidences of overall mortality in patients implanted with SES and treated with BA after first TLR
SES indicates sirolimus-eluting stent; BA, balloon angioplasty; and TLR, target lesion

revascularization.
Figure 3
Cumulative incidences of second TLR in patients implanted with SES and treated with BA

SES indicates sirolimus-eluting stent; BA, balloon angioplasty; and TLR, target lesion revascularization.
Figure 4
Cumulative incidences of stent thrombosis in patients implanted with SES and treated with BA after first TLR

SES indicates sirolimus-eluting stent; BA, balloon angioplasty; and TLR, target lesion revascularization.

Figure 1

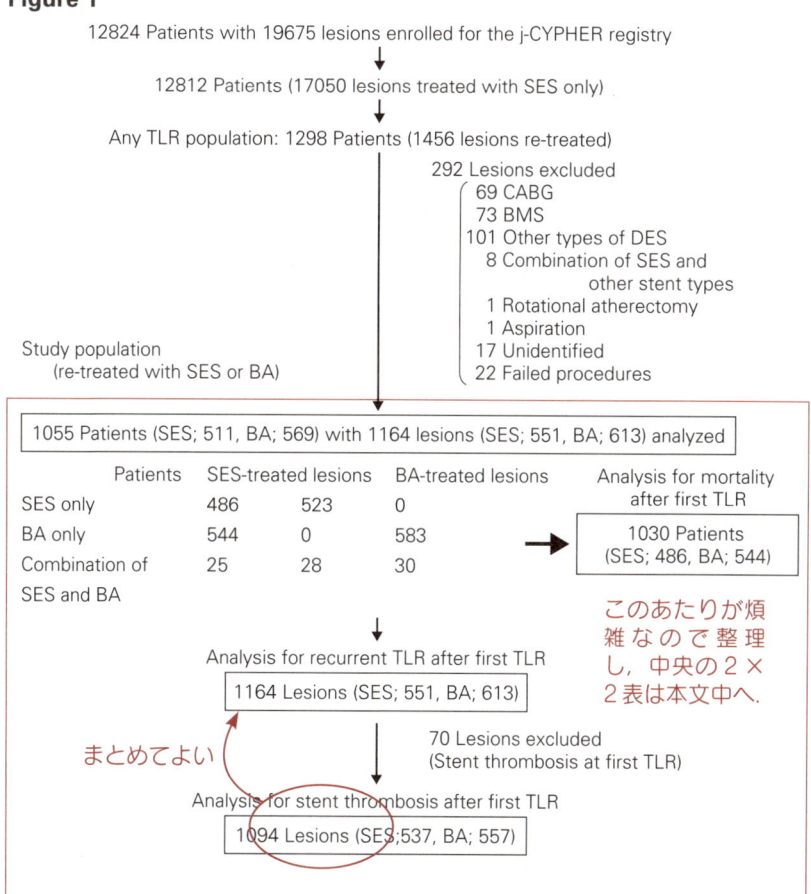

12824 Patients with 19675 lesions enrolled for the j-CYPHER registry
↓
12812 Patients (17050 lesions treated with SES only)
↓
Any TLR population: 1298 Patients (1456 lesions re-treated)

292 Lesions excluded
- 69 CABG
- 73 BMS
- 101 Other types of DES
- 8 Combination of SES and other stent types
- 1 Rotational atherectomy
- 1 Aspiration
- 17 Unidentified
- 22 Failed procedures

Study population (re-treated with SES or BA)
↓

1055 Patients (SES; 511, BA; 569) with 1164 lesions (SES; 551, BA; 613) analyzed

	Patients	SES-treated lesions	BA-treated lesions
SES only	486	523	0
BA only	544	0	583
Combination of SES and BA	25	28	30

Analysis for mortality after first TLR
1030 Patients (SES; 486, BA; 544)

↓
Analysis for recurrent TLR after first TLR
1164 Lesions (SES; 551, BA; 613)
↓
70 Lesions excluded (Stent thrombosis at first TLR)
↓
Analysis for stent thrombosis after first TLR
1094 Lesions (SES;537, BA; 557)

このあたりが煩雑なので整理し，中央の２×２表は本文中へ．

まとめてよい

143

Figure 2

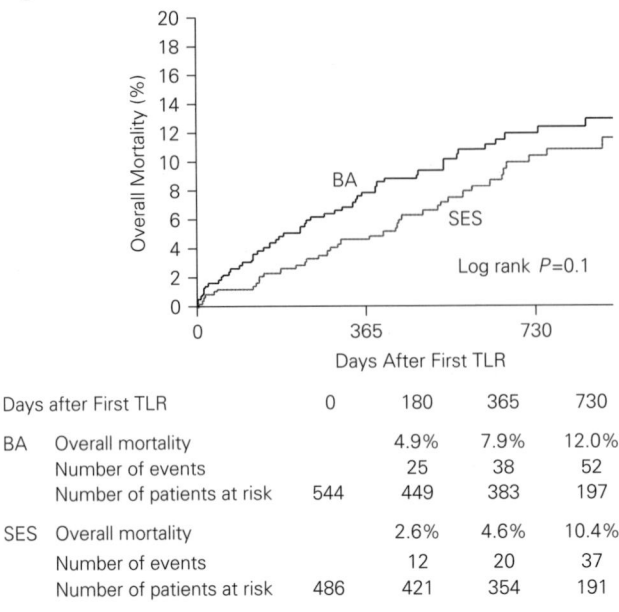

Days after First TLR	0	180	365	730
BA Overall mortality		4.9%	7.9%	12.0%
Number of events		25	38	52
Number of patients at risk	544	449	383	197
SES Overall mortality		2.6%	4.6%	10.4%
Number of events		12	20	37
Number of patients at risk	486	421	354	191

Figure 3

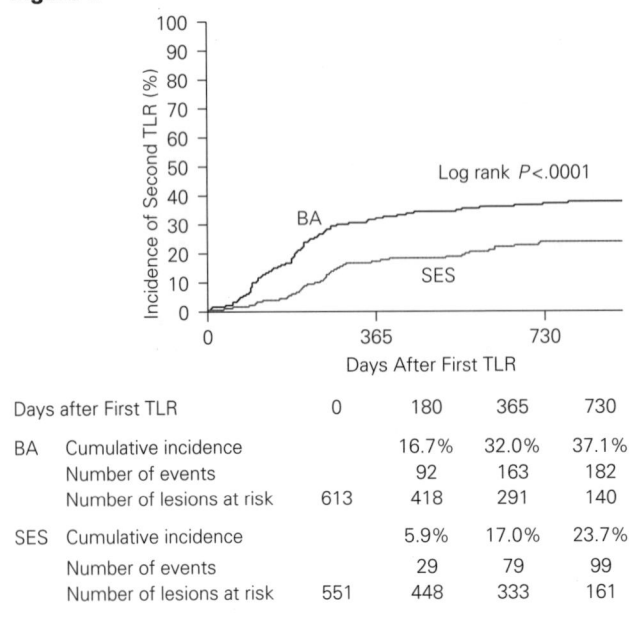

Days after First TLR	0	180	365	730
BA Cumulative incidence		16.7%	32.0%	37.1%
Number of events		92	163	182
Number of lesions at risk	613	418	291	140
SES Cumulative incidence		5.9%	17.0%	23.7%
Number of events		29	79	99
Number of lesions at risk	551	448	333	161

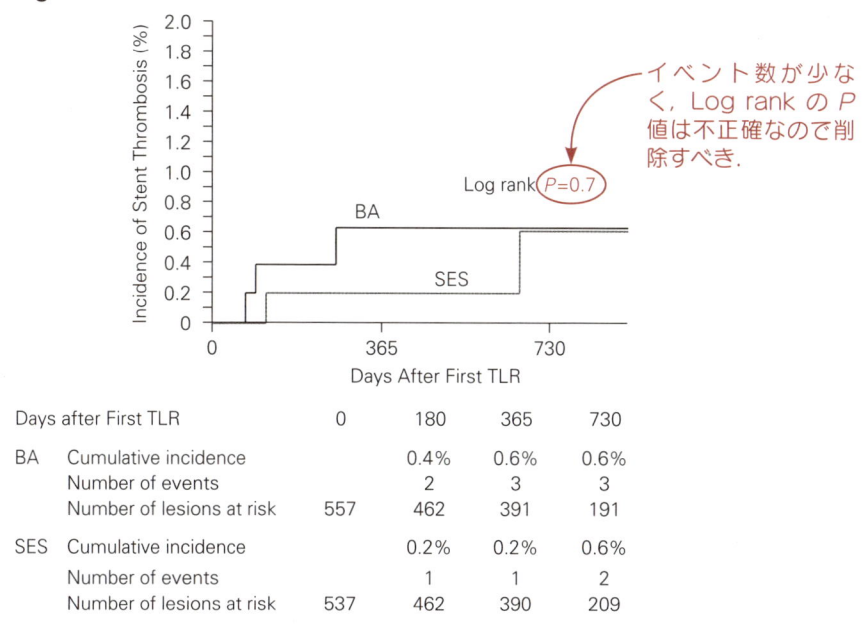

Figure 4

[Graph: Incidence of Stent Thrombosis (%) vs Days After First TLR, showing BA and SES curves with "Log rank P=0.7" annotation]

イベント数が少なく，Log rank の P 値は不正確なので削除すべき．

Days after First TLR		0	180	365	730
BA	Cumulative incidence		0.4%	0.6%	0.6%
	Number of events		2	3	3
	Number of lesions at risk	557	462	391	191
SES	Cumulative incidence		0.2%	0.2%	0.6%
	Number of events		1	1	2
	Number of lesions at risk	537	462	390	209

4編　表現は明確に／結論は結果から導き出される主たるメッセージ

Table 1. Baseline Patient Characteristics

Characteristics	SES (n=486)	BA (n=544)	P Value
Age, y	67.5 ± 10.2	67.6 ± 10.1	0.8
Age >=80 y	49 (10%)	56 (10%)	0.9
Male	373 (77%)	427 (78%)	0.5
Body mass index	23.7 ± 3.5	23.9 ± 3.3	0.5
Body mass index >=25.0	167 (34%)	186 (34%)	1.0
Hypertension	369 (76%)	413 (76%)	1.0
Diabetes mellitus	230 (47%)	306 (56%)	0.004
Insulin therapy	63 (13%)	107 (20%)	0.004
Current smoking	90 (19%)	100 (18%)	1.0
Treatment for hypercholesterolemia	218 (45%)	254 (47%)	0.6
Serum creatinine	1.86 ± 2.61	2.18 ± 3.08	0.07
eGFR (mL/min/1.73m^2)	56.4 ± 27.7	52.3 ± 27.4	0.02
eGFR<30, without hemodialysis	24 (6%)	30 (6%)	0.6
Hemodialysis	61 (13%)	82 (15%)	0.2
Acute Coronary Syndrome	113 (23%)	111 (20%)	0.3
ST-elevation myocardial infarction	46 (9%)	32 (6%)	0.03
Non-STEMI	10 (2%)	11 (2%)	1.0
Unstable angina pectoris	57 (12%)	68 (13%)	0.7
Prior myocardial infarction	139 (29%)	168 (31%)	0.4
Prior stroke	53 (11%)	54 (10%)	0.6
Peripheral vascular disease	82 (17%)	72 (13%)	0.1
Prior heart failure	62 (13%)	62 (11%)	0.5
Diseased vessels			
Single-vessel disease	168 (35%)	205 (38%)	0.3
Double-vessel disease	138 (28%)	151 (28%)	0.8
Triple-vessel disease	84 (17%)	82 (15%)	0.3
Unprotected LMCA	36 (7%)	57 (10%)	0.09
Prior CABG	60 (12%)	49 (9%)	0.08
Ejection Fraction (%)	57.4 ± 13.6	55.4 ± 13.6	0.03
Ejection fraction =<40%	56 (12%)	62 (11%)	1.0
Emergent procedure	44 (9%)	42 (8%)	0.4

SES indicates sirolimus-eluting stent; BA, balloon angioplasty; eGFR, estimated glomerular filtration rate; non STEMI, non-ST-elevation myocardial infarction; LMCA, left main coronary artery; and CABG, coronary artery bypass grafting.

大文字で始まる単語とそうでない単語があって不統一．投稿雑誌をみて合わせる．

％はどこかにまとめて示せばよく，このように各行に書くと煩雑．

Table 2. Lesion and Procedural Characteristics

	SES (n=551)	BA (n=613)	P Value
Lesion location			
LAD	235 (43%)	229 (37%)	0.07
LCx	66 (12%)	114 (19%)	0.002
RCA	206 (37%)	223 (36%)	0.7
LMCA	22 (4%)	38 (6%)	0.09
Saphenous vein graft	20 (4%)	7 (1%)	0.004
De novo lesion	400 (73%)	401 (65%)	0.008
In-stent restenosis	81 (15%)	154 (25%)	<0.0001
STEMI culprit lesion	23 (4%)	17 (3%)	0.2
Ostial location	64 (12%)	93 (15%)	0.08
Chronic total occlusion	60 (11%)	85 (14%)	0.1
Severe calcification	84 (15%)	99 (16%)	0.7
Bifurcation lesion	123 (22%)	158 (26%)	0.2
Side branch stenting	34 (6%)	65 (11%)	0.006
Complex lesion (B2&C)	433 (79%)	502 (82%)	0.2
Lesion length >=30 mm	128 (23%)	178 (29%)	0.03
Preprocedural reference diameter <2.5 mm	171 (31%)	193 (31%)	0.9
Use of intravascular ultrasound	264 (48%)	244 (40%)	0.005
Direct stenting	100 (18%)	68 (11%)	0.0006
Additional dilatation	272 (49%)	308 (50%)	0.8
Maximum inflation pressure, atm	18.2±3.5	18.5±3.4	0.2
No. of stents used	1.5±0.7	1.6±0.8	0.0004
Length of stents used, mm	33.9±19.3	37.9±21.5	0.001
Minimal stent size, mm	2.86±0.35	2.79±0.35	0.002

SES indicates sirolimus-eluting stent; BA, balloon angioplasty; LAD, left anterior descending coronary artery; LCx, left circumflex coronary artery; RCA, right coronary artery; LMCA, left main coronary artery; and STEMI, ST-elevation myocardial infarction.

Table 3. Univariate Correlates of Second Target Lesion Revascularization Within One Year

Variables	Second TLR Yes (n=242)	Second TLR No (n=624)	P Value
SES implantation	79 (33%)	333 (53%)	<0.0001
Age >=80 y	26 (11%)	50 (8%)	0.2
Male	187 (77%)	483 (77%)	1.0
Body mass index >=25.0	70 (29%)	223 (36%)	0.06
Hypertension	182 (75%)	471 (75%)	0.9
Diabetes mellitus	137 (57%)	337 (54%)	0.5
Insulin therapy	50 (21%)	110 (18%)	0.3
Current smoking	38 (16%)	117 (19%)	0.3
Treatment for hypercholesterolemia	122 (50%)	286 (46%)	0.2
eGFR<30, without hemodialysis	16 (7%)	24 (4%)	0.09
Hemodialysis	47 (19%)	70 (11%)	0.002
Acute coronary syndrome	55 (23%)	133 (21%)	0.7
Prior myocardial infarction	60 (25%)	170 (27%)	0.5
Prior stroke	28 (12%)	64 (10%)	0.6
Peripheral vascular disease	36 (15%)	86 (14%)	0.7
Prior heart failure	40 (17%)	69 (11%)	0.03
Diseased vessels			
Single vessel disease	79 (33%)	205 (33%)	1.0
Double vessel disease	61 (25%)	192 (31%)	0.1
Triple vessel disease	50 (21%)	106 (17%)	0.2
Unprotected LMCA	28 (12%)	58 (9%)	0.3
Prior CABG	24 (10%)	63 (10%)	0.9
Ejection fraction =<40%	30 (12%)	66 (11%)	0.5
Emergent procedure	25 (10%)	53 (8%)	0.4
Lesion location			
LAD	86 (36%)	251 (40%)	0.2
LCx	41 (17%)	88 (14%)	0.3
RCA	95 (39%)	234 (38%)	0.6
LMCA	12 (5%)	35 (6%)	0.7
Saphenous vein graft	7 (3%)	14 (2%)	0.6
De novo lesion	150 (62%)	435 (70%)	0.03
In-stent restenosis	64 (26%)	118 (19%)	0.02
STEMI culprit lesion	4 (2%)	28 (4%)	0.03
Ostial location	34 (14%)	84 (13%)	0.8
Chronic total occlusion	29 (12%)	76 (12%)	0.9
Severe calcification	53 (22%)	91 (15%)	0.01
Bifurcation lesion	60 (25%)	149 (24%)	0.8
Side branch stenting	22 (9%)	51 (8%)	0.7
Complex lesion (B2&C)	198 (82%)	505 (81%)	0.8
Lesion length >=30 mm	72 (30%)	162 (26%)	0.3
Preprocedural reference diameter <2.5 mm	73 (30%)	193 (31%)	0.8
Use of intravascular ultrasound	92 (38%)	292 (47%)	0.02
Direct stenting	17 (7%)	88 (14%)	0.003
Additional dilatation	115 (48%)	324 (52%)	0.2

TLR indicates target lesion revascularization; SES, sirolimus-eluting stent; eGFR, estimated glomerular filtration rate; LMCA, left main coronary artery; CABG, coronary artery bypass grafting; LAD, left anterior descending coronary artery; LCx, left circumflex coronary artery; RCA, right coronary artery; and STEMI, ST-elevation myocardial infarction.

Table 4. Sirolimus-Eluting Stents in Comparison With Balloon Aagioplasty for Treatment of Sirolimus-Eluting Stent Restenosis

Variables	Univariate Odds Ratio (95% CI)	Multivariate Odds Ratio (95% CI)	P Value
SES-implantation (vs. BA)	0.42 (0.31 to 0.58)	0.45 (0.33 to 0.63)	<0.001
Hemodialysis	1.91 (1.27 to 2.85)	1.61 (1.02 to 2.52)	0.04
Prior heart failure	1.59 (1.04 to 2.42)	1.41 (0.89 to 2.19)	0.1
De novo lesion	0.71 (0.52 to 0.97)	0.93 (0.57 to 1.54)	0.8
In-stent restenosis	1.54 (1.08 to 2.18)	1.19 (0.68 to 2.09)	0.5
ST-elevation myocardial infarction culprit lesion	0.36 (0.11 to 0.92)	0.40 (0.12 to 1.07)	0.07
Severe calcification	1.64 (1.12 to 2.39)	1.39 (0.91 to 2.10)	0.1
Use of intravascular ultrasound	0.70 (0.51 to 0.94)	0.80 (0.58 to 1.10)	0.2
Direct stenting	0.46 (0.26 to 0.77)	0.63 (0.35 to 1.08)	0.09

CI indicates confidence intervals; SES, sirolimus-eluting stent; and BA, balloon angioplasty.

本編のAfter論文は出版社の許諾が下りなかったため，掲載しておりません．

5編 「何を言いたいのか」が不明な記述をしない 具体的な数字を入れる

Before

COMPLETE CESSATION OF IMMUNOSUPPRESSION AFTER PEDIATRIC LIVING DONOR LIVER TRANSPLANTATION

FOOTNOTE

ABSTRACT

(background)
Successful establishment of operational tolerance (complete cessation of IS), albeit representing the ultimate goal in transplant (Tx) medicine, has been difficult to be attempted due to the risk of rejection. In the setting of our living-donor liver transplantation (LDLT), feasibility and safety of operational tolerance were evaluated. In addition, relevant clinical predictors of operational tolerance were explored.

(Method)
In pediatric LDLT, IS was weaned off either by our elective protocol (electively) or forcibly discontinued due to severe complications of IS or noncompliance (non-electively). Protocol biopsy was performed on a subset of the patients either free from IS or during the weaning process. In addition, whether and how several clinical parameters correlate with successful IS withdrawal were investigated using univariate and multivariable analyses.

(Results)
Out of 675 patients who underwent LDLT, 191 patients were

この論文は論文を書き始めたばかりの著者が，一番最初に書いた初稿である．最終掲載論文と大きく異なるが，これから論文を初めて書こうとする若手研究者の参考例とする．

そもそも行間が狭く，人に見てもらう論文になっていない（注：ダブルスペースになっていなかった）．

このパラグラフ全体の目的が不明．免疫抑制剤の完全中止が移植のゴールに思えてしまう．

①この単語の意味が不明．

研究方法，デザインが不明．

②突然，多変量解析が出てくる．

assessed for weaning IS, either electively or non-electively. 85 patients (45%) were completely weaned off IS, while only 22 patients (12%) exhibited clinical sign of rejection, which was successfully counteracted by an increase of tacrolimus or corticosteroid pulse therapy. 26 patients (14%) resumed minimal maintenance IS due to the presence of graft fibrosis detected by protocol biopsy. 56 patients (29%) were still undergoing weaning IS. 2 patiensts (1%) resumed full maintenance IS due to de novo AIH. Among several clinical parameters, the presence of HLA-B mismatch between donors and recipients (OR=33.36, p=0.05) and the absence of early rejection episode (OR= p=0.002) were statistically significant predictors of successful IS withdrawal. OR of Female donor reached as high as 5.32, although its p value was 0.16.

(Conclusion)
Significantly higher proportion (45%) of all the patients assessed for weaning IS, compared with those of other transplant centers achieved operational tolerance. On the other hand, any immunological penalty such as graft loss has never been encountered during weaning process. The presence of HLA-B mismatch between donors and recipients and the absence of early rejection episode were statistically significant predictors of successful IS withdrawal

*

METHODS

Pediatric LDLT

675 pediatric patients underwent LDLT at Kyoto University Hospital from June 1990 and April 2008. All the patients underwent standard LDLT. All the graft were flushed and preserved with histidine-tryptophan-ketoglutarate (HTK) solution. All the LDLTs were performed by the Kyoto method as described previously ( ).

Immunosuppression (IS)

In our current protocol, the baseline IS regimen consisted of tacrolimus and low-dose steroids. Tacrolimus was administered twice a day orally from pre-transplant day 1, except the cases of hepatic encephalopathy or infection. The target trough level of tacrolimus was 10 to 15 ng/mL for the first 2 weeks, followed by 5 to 10 ng/mL for following 2 months. After discharge, the dose of tacrolimus was determined individually depending on each patient's condition.

The initial steroid was methylprednisolone, which was intravenously administered at a dosage of 10mg/kg immediately after perfusion, followed by a dosage of 1mg/kg twice daily for the first 3 days, 0.5mg/kg twice daily for the next 3 days, and 0.3mg/kg on day 7. From day 8, predonisolone was started to be given orally at a dosage of 0.3mg/kg/day, which was gradually tapered and then was stopped in 3 months As far as the first 60 cases are concerned, unlike the subsequent cases, induction IS therapy was performed by the administration of continuous intravenous high-dose tacrolimus within the 1st week post-Tx, In those cases, tacrolimus levels were as high as 40 to 50 ng/mL and they were not comparable with those in the subsequent cases. Therefore, they were excluded from the analysis .

IS withdrawal (Fig1)

IS withdrawal was initiated by the physician-controlled IS weaning protocol (protocol weaning off IS) or the management of post-Tx infection (cholangitis, Epstein-Barr virus [EBV], hepatitis B virus [HBV] or PTLD, or as a result of patient non-compliance (non-protocol)). Outlines of IS weaning protocol are described in Fig1. IS weaning protocol was started when patients satisfy the following criteria : (1) pediatric recipient; (2) 2 years post-Tx; (3) no single episode of rejection during the preceding 12 months;(4) a normal liver function. Informed consent was provided according to the declaration of Helsinki . Parental permission was obtained for patients who were younger than 20 years of ages . All of them entered this study after giving their fully informed consent. For the forcibly weaned patients, tacrolumus was weaned depending on the individual patient's clinical course.

Diagnosis Monitoring and treatment of for acute rejection

During the weaning process or after cessation of IS, the patients were carefully monitored by transamynases for rejection. When an increase in transamynases was observed, the dosage of tacrolimus was increased or corticosteroid pulse therapy was administered with or without histology. Acute rejection was diagnosed clinically on the basis of an increase in aspartate aminotransferase (AST) and alanine aminotransferase (ALT) or gamma glutamyl transpeptidase (γ GTP), or all three, with or without histological evidence. Histologic diagnosis and grading of acute rejection were performed according to the criteria proposed by Demetris et al. We treated the rejection with a steroid bolus injection (10mg/kg) or the resumption of IS. We used additional immunosuppressants, such as OKT3 to steroid-resistant rejection, which was defined as a refractory rejection even after several course of steroid injection. Additional immunosuppressants such as OKT3 were used to counteract steroid-resistant rejection.

Protocol biopsy Diagnosis and treatment of fibrosis

Since January 2003, protocol biopsy has been performed on our pediatric patients 1,2,5 and 10 years post-Tx, despite normal liver test. It has demonstrated that fibrosis is present in a portal area in a subset of the IS free patients in a greater extent, compared with the patients on maintenance IS. The degree of fibrosis has been quantified following the Ishak's modified staging on Masson trichrome stained section. At present it remains elusive whether fibrosis present in the IS free patients would be antigen-dependent, since time between Tx and protocol biopsy has been significantly longer in IS free patients than that in maintenance IS However, IS was reintroduced in the IS free patients or increased in the patients in the weaning process, in case that advanced fibrosis (bridging fibrosis) was observed by single biopsy or progression of fibrosis was proven by repeated biopsy ( ).

Fibrosis was usually diagnosed by protocol biopsy after transplantation. In most of the cases AST, ALT or γGTP were normal. We checked blood flow carefully by Doppler echo and CT scan. If we found the obstruction of hepatic vein or portal vein, we dilated it by intravenous technique.

But to the other patients we resumed IS for the moment without the evidence of rejection and performed follow-up biopsy every year.

Genetic typing

Haplotypes were serologically defined for HLA-A, HLA-B and HLA-DR loci in donors and recipients except emergency LDLT for fulminant hepatitis.

Because all the recipients were pediatric and received grafts from their biological parents, the donors and the recipients were either haplo-identical or identical at each HLA loci. Therefore, they have only one or no mismatched allele for each locus.

Analysis to evaluate correlation between successful IS withdrawal and clinical parameters.

①Depending on whether at 10 years post-Tx, the patients were completely free from IS for more than 1 year, or on maintenance IS due to the experience of rejection during the weaning process or after cessation of IS, the patients were devided into tolerance

①重要なアウトカムの定義であり、わかりやすく示すと同時に、Methodsの前のほうにもっていく.

group (Gr-Tol) and intolerance group (Gr-Intol).② We compared this two groups in following clinical parameters:. Two groups were compared with respect to following clinical parameters; recipient/donor age, recipient/donor gender, ABO compatibility, ABO incompatibility, HLA-A/HLA-B/HLA-DR mismatch, graft weight (GRBW%), average trough level of tacrolimus (ng/mL) within the 1st week post-Tx and rejection episode in the 1st month-Tx.③ As far as the first 60 cases are concerned, unlike the subsequent cases, induction IS therapy was performed by the administration of continuous intravenous high-dose tacrolimus within the 1st week post-Tx, In those cases, tacrolimus levels were as high as 40 to 50 ng/mL and they were not comparable with those in the subsequent cases (10 to 12 ng/mL). Therefore, they were excluded from the analysis.

④ [In this study, we compared two status groups at 10 years after LDLTx. One is consisted of 50 patients who are free from IS for more than 1 year (Gol-off). The other is consisted of 13 patients who have had rejection episode and have resumed IS in weaning course (Gol-rej)]

⑤ We used univariate analyses (T test for continuous variables and chi-square or Fishier's exact tests for dichotomous variables) and multivariable analyses (Logistic regression model).

② 大雑把すぎる．何を2群間で比較したのか？この場合，アウトカムがわかっているので背景因子（何々と明示）について比較することを記載．

③ 解析の後ろに突然免疫抑制のプロトコルが出ている．プロトコルはどこかにまとめる．

④ 対象患者の数に関することはできるだけResultsに．

⑤ multivariable analyses では何をしたか不明．

RESULTS

The out come of weaning (Fig2)

Out of 675 patients, 484 patients (71.7%) either did not satisfy the aforementioned criteria of the weaning protocol because of their unstable liver function or were not assessed for IS weaning process solely beacuse cooperation of local physicians who followed the patients was not available.

a) Elective weaning

142 patients (21.0%) satisfied the criteria and were assessed for IS weaning. Out of them, 64 patients (45%) successfully stop IS. Only 6 patients (4%) experienced rejection either during weaning process or after complete cessation of IS. 56 patients (39%) are undergoing weaning IS. Out of 64 patients who once had stopped IS, 8 patients resumed IS due to the presence of graft fibrosis, despite normal liver test. As a consequence, 56 patients are IS free at present. In 15 patients who had been in weaning process, IS was increased due to presence of graft fibrosis. 1 patient failed to stop IS due to de novo AIH.

because が2つ続いて読みにくい．定義はMethodsで書くので，ここでは何人（％）がどうなったと明確に記載．

できるだけ図を使って解析集団がわかるようにする．また表を使って解析された集団と除外された集団とを比較し，対象集団の特徴を明確にする．

b) Non-elective weaning

49 patients (7.3%) stopped IS because of life-threatening complications (PTLD, EBV infection, HBV infection, cholangitis etc) or non-compliance. Out of them, 31 patients (63%) successfully stopped IS. 16 patients (33%) experienced rejection. 2 patients resumed IS due to the presence of graft fibrosis, despite normal liver test. At present, 29 patients are free from IS. 1 patient failed to stop IS due to de novo AIH.

c) Rejection

At present, altogether 85 patients (56+29) (12.6%) are IS free while 22 patients (6+16) experienced rejection during the weaning process or after cessation of IS. The average time between the start of weaning and the cessation of IS was 41.3 months (ranging from 0 to 120.9 months) and the average of IS free period was 83.8 months (ranging from 12.2 to 161.8 months)

Correlation between successful cessation of IS and clinical parameters

Since as described in Methods, subjects of analyses were selected depending on whether at 10 years post-Tx, the patients were IS free or not. Out of 85 IS free patients, 50 patients were included into the analysis (Gr-Tol), while out of 22 rejection experienced patients, 13 patients were included into the analysis (Gr-Intol).

The results of univariate analysis are shown in table1. Univariate analyses revealed that there were no significant differences between Gr-Tol and Gr-Intol with respect to recipient/donor age, recipient gender, ABO compatibility, ABO incompatibility, HLA-A/HLA-B/HLA-DR mismatch, graft weight (GRBW%) or average trough level of tacrolimus within the 1st week post-Tx. Of note, in Gr-Tol, 77% patients received their graft from biological mother while in Gr-Intol, that is the case in 38% (Gr-Tol and Gr-Intol; 77% and. 38%, P=0.01). In addition, Gol-Intol had experienced rejection within 1month post-Tx at a significantly higher incidence than Gr-Tol (Gr-Tol and Gr-Intol; 10%,and 69% P<0.001).

At the next step, multivariable analysis was used to determine whether there was correlation between successful IS cessation and HLA-A/HLA-B/HLA-DR mismatch, in addition to donor gender and early post-Tx rejection episode which had been revealed by univariate analysis to be candidates associated with successful IS withdrawal. Since linkage between HLA matching and successful IS cessation had been suggested by our earlier study, multivariable analysis included matching of each HLA loci (　). The results of multivariable analysis were shown in Fig3. Among the individual parameters tested herein, multivariable logistic model revealed that the presence of HLA-B mismatch, the absence of HLA-A mismatch and the absence of early rejection episode (< 1month post-Tx) were statistically significant positive predictors of successful cessation of IS (the presence of HLA –B mismatch; OR 33.36, p=0.05, the absence of HLA-A mismatch; p=0.091, the absence of early rejection episode; p=0.002). As far as female donor was concerned, OR reached as high as 5.32, although the difference between Gr-Tol and Gr-Intol did not reach significance.

多変量解析の結果は表にしたほうがわかりやすい．

＊

＊Discussion がない．

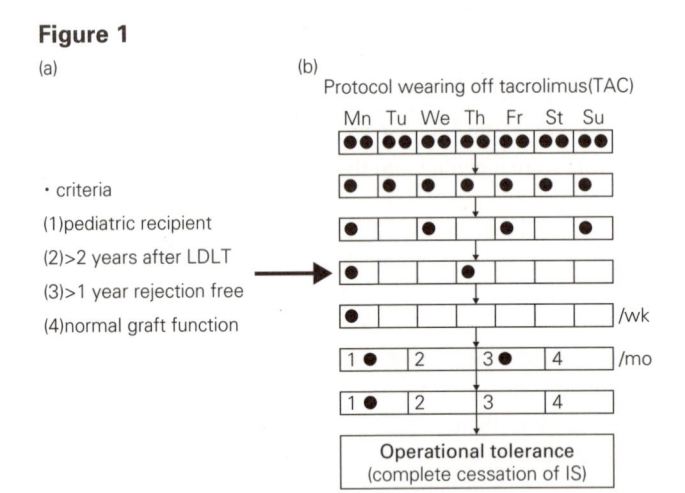

Figure 1

(a)
・criteria
(1)pediatric recipient
(2)>2 years after LDLT
(3)>1 year rejection free
(4)normal graft function

(b) Protocol wearing off tacrolimus(TAC)

Figure 2

Outcome of Weaning (June, 1990- April, 2008)

540 surviving pediatric patients

論文では 675 とあるのに，そこからスタートしないのはおかしい．

191 assessed as weaning
-142 protocol IS weaning
-49 non-elective IS off

349 out of the criteria or not assessed as weaning

65 protocol IS weaning
38 non-elective IS off

21 protocol IS weaning
11 non-elective IS off

103 operational tolerance

excluded
-53 <10 years from LDLT

50 Tolerance group

32 Resumed IS
-14 rejection
-2 AIH
-16 fibrosis

excluded
-1 rejection (< 10 years from LDLT)
-2 AIH
-16 fibrosis

13 Intolerance group

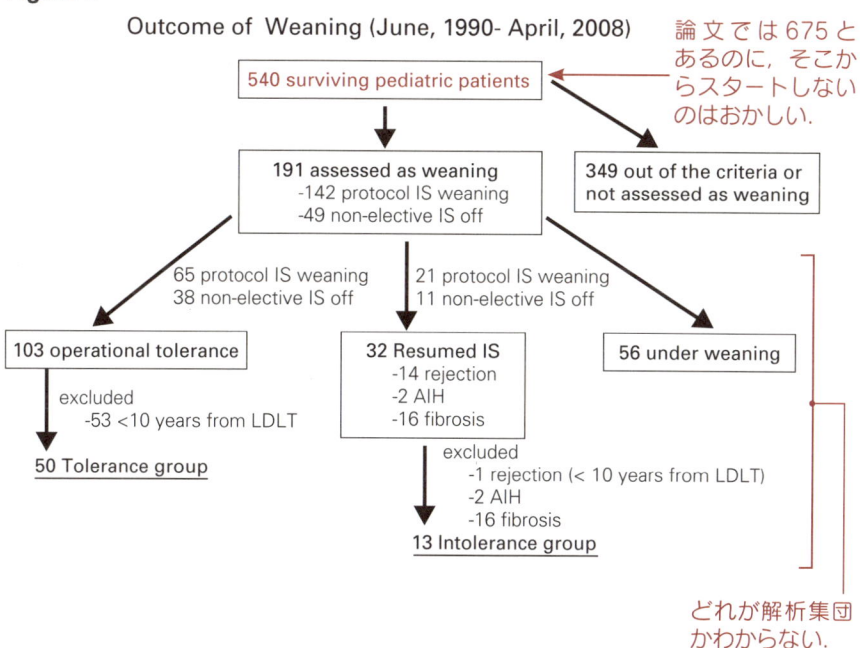

56 under weaning

どれが解析集団かわからない．

Figure 3

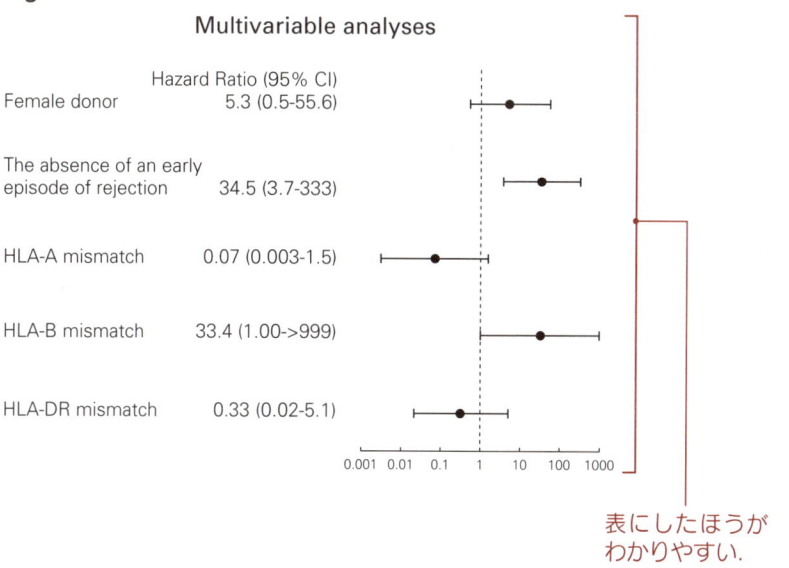

Multivariable analyses

	Hazard Ratio (95% CI)
Female donor	5.3 (0.5-55.6)
The absence of an early episode of rejection	34.5 (3.7-333)
HLA-A mismatch	0.07 (0.003-1.5)
HLA-B mismatch	33.4 (1.00->999)
HLA-DR mismatch	0.33 (0.02-5.1)

0.001 0.01 0.1 1 10 100 1000

表にしたほうがわかりやすい．

Table1
Univariate analysis
Status at 10 years after LDLT

	Tolerance group	Intolerance group	
	N=50	N=13	p-value
Recipient age, mean (SD)	2y11m (6.7m)	3y1m (14.1m)	0.92
Donor age, mean (SD)	32.2 (0.8)	31.8 (2.7)	0.89
Recipient female, N (%)	33 (66%)	11 (85%)	0.31
Donor female, N (%)	31 (62%)	3 (23%)	0.01
ABO compatible, N (%)	15 (30%)	3 (23%)	0.74
ABO incompatible, N (%)	2 (4%)	2 (15%)	0.19
HLA-A mismatch, N (%)	32 (72%)	8 (80%)	0.99
HLA-B mismatch, N (%)	41 (93%)	8 (80%)	0.23
HLA-DR mismatch, N (%)	36 (82%)	8 (80%)	0.99
Graft weight (GRBW%), mean (SD)	3.02 (0.20)	3.11 (0.41)	0.83
Tacrolimus trough level (ng/ml), mean (SD) (average within the 1st week post-LDLT)	11.53(0.71)	12.51(1.31)	0.5
The early episode of rejection, N (%) (<1st month post-LDLT)	5 (10%)	9 (69%)	<0.0001

Donor と Recipient の情報は交互にこないように，まとめて記載．

月齢を混ぜないように．

Transplant International ISSN 0934-0874

ORIGINAL ARTICLE

Factors affecting operational tolerance after pediatric living-donor liver transplantation: impact of early post-transplant events and HLA match*

Hidenori Ohe,[1]** Kayo Waki,[2,3] Mami Yoshitomi,[1] Takeshi Morimoto,[4] Hanaa Nafady-Hego,[1,5] Naoki Satoda,[1] Ying Li,[1] Xiangdong Zhao,[1] Shimon Sakaguchi,[6] Shinji Uemoto,[1] G. Alex Bishop[7] and Takaaki Koshiba[8]

1 Department of Surgery, Graduate School of Medicine, Kyoto University, Kyoto, Japan
2 Graduate School of Medicine, University of Tokyo, Department of Diabetes and Metabolic Diseases, Tokyo, Japan
3 Graduate School of Medicine, University of Tokyo, Department of Ubiquitous Health Informatics, Tokyo, Japan
4 Center for Medical Education and Clinical Epidemiology Unit, Graduate School of Medicine, Kyoto University, Kyoto, Japan
5 Department of Microbiology and Immunology, Graduate School of Medicine, Assiut University, Assiut, Egypt
6 World Premier International Research Center, Immunology Frontier Research Center, Osaka University, Osaka, Japan
7 Transplantation Laboratory, Royal Prince Alfred Hospital, Sydney, Australia
8 Department of Biology, Molecular Pharmacology, Graduate School of Science, Kobe University, Kobe, Japan

Keywords
HLA, living-donor liver transplantation, operational tolerance, pediatric.

Correspondence
Takaaki Koshiba MD, PhD, Department of Biology, Molecular Pharmacology, Graduate School of Science, Kobe University, Rokkodaicho 1-1, Nada-ku, Kobe 657-8501, Japan.
Tel./fax: +81-75-211-8780; e-mail: tkoshiba@port.kobe-u.ac.jp

Conflicts of Interest
All authors have no potential interest to declare.

*Part of this work was presented at the 15th Congress of the European Society for Organ Transplantation held in Glasgow, UK, 4–7 September 2011 and at the American Transplant Congress, April 30–May 4, 2011, PA, USA

**This work was supported by the ATC International Young Investigator Award (2011) (H.O.).

Received: 4 June 2011
Revision requested: 11 July 2011
Accepted: 25 October 2011
Published online: 26 November 2011

doi:10.1111/j.1432-2277.2011.01389.x

Summary

Pediatric recipients of living-donor liver transplants (LDLT) can often discontinue immunosuppression (IS). We examined factors affecting development of operational tolerance (OT), defined as off IS for >1 year, in this population. A historic cohort analysis was conducted in 134 pediatric primary semi-allogeneic LDLT. Multivariate logistic regression analysis was used. The frequency of peripheral regulatory T cells (Tregs) was determined at >10 years post-Tx by FACS analysis. IS was successfully discontinued in 84 tolerant patients (Gr-tol), but not in 50 intolerant patients (Gr-intol). The Gr-intol consisted of 24 patients with rejection (Gr-rej) and 26 with fibrosis of grafts (Gr-fib). The absence of early rejection [odds ratio (OR) 2.79, 95% CI 1.11–7.02, $P = 0.03$], was a positive independent predictor, whereas HLA-A mismatch (0.18, 0.03–0.91, $P = 0.04$) was a negative predictor. HLA-DR mismatches did not affect OT. The Treg frequency was significantly decreased in Gr-intol (4.9%) compared with Gr-tol (7.6%) ($P = 0.003$). There were increased levels of tacrolimus in the first week in Gr-Tol ($P = 0.02$). Although HLA-B mismatch (8.73, 1.09–70.0, $P = 0.04$) was a positive independent predictor of OT, its clinical significance remains doubtful. In this large cohort of pediatric LDLT recipients, absence of early rejection, HLA-A match and the later predominance of Tregs are factors associated with OT.

Introduction

Living-donor liver transplantation (LDLT) has become a standard approach to save lives of patients suffering from end-stage liver disease [1]. There has been a rapid increase in the number of living-donor transplants (Tx) for both liver and kidney because of the shortage of deceased donors. One problem that has remained unsolved is the dependency of the patients on nonspecific life-long immunosuppression (IS) accompanied by complications [2]. Therefore, the establishment of operational tolerance (OT) in a proportion of liver Tx patients provides an opportunity to assess factors that promote tolerance [3–6]. For the following analysis, we have defined OT as continued function of a transplanted organ in the absence of IS with a follow up of >1 year.

Although immunomodulatory strategies efficiently induce tolerance in animals, tolerance after clinical organ Tx is most unusual [7–14]. However, we have developed an elective protocol that enables a substantial proportion of selected LDLT patients to be weaned off IS [15]. Some patients who stopped IS nonelectively because of infection, severe side effects or noncompliance, but did not exhibit any clinical manifestation of rejection, were included [15]. Altogether, OT occurred in 15% of all pediatric patients, regardless of whether IS was weaned electively or nonelectively, comparable with other Tx centers [16,17]. Thus, the strategy for weaning from IS has been very successful, providing a large patient cohort to investigate mechanisms of OT [18–21]. The patient cohort in this study consists of parental donors to child recipients (parent to F1). In most recipients, this led to a one haplotype difference at all HLA loci (referred to here as mismatched), except where both the mother and the father shared the same HLA allele at a particular locus. Tx in these individuals were matched at these loci (referred to here as matched).

There is considerable interest currently as to whether complete cessation of IS in the setting of pediatric LDLT is the most appropriate approach for these patients. Thus, we have investigated this population to identify factors that contribute to OT. In marked contrast to renal Tx, for which the overall survival is better when there are fewer donor–recipient HLA mismatches, HLA matching does not affect the overall survival of deceased donor liver Tx [22–28]. Nonetheless, to our knowledge, only limited data are available on the significance of HLA matches in the development of OT after liver Tx. Two reports showed that more HLA matches were associated with the development of OT after deceased donor liver Tx [29,30]. Consequently, one of the factors used in our analysis was HLA match. Previous studies from our group showed that patients who have been removed from IS can develop advanced or progressing graft fibrosis, often associated with deposition of C4d [31]. As this fibrosis often improves with re-introduction of IS [32], patients with fibrosis who recommenced IS were included in the intolerant group.

Research design and methods

Study design, statistical analysis, and population

This was a historic cohort analysis based on 670 pediatric patients who underwent LDLT at Kyoto University Hospital from June 1990 to April 2008. All operations were performed by the Kyoto method [33]. OT patients (Group-tolerance – Gr-tol) were defined as stable normal graft function for more than 1 year off IS [3–6]. On the other hand, failure to discontinue IS because of rejection (Gr-rej) or fibrosis (Gr-fib) during the process of weaning IS or after cessation of IS were referred to as intolerance (Group-intolerance – Gr-intol) [15,31]. We compared baseline characteristics of Gr-rej with Gr-fib using the t-test for continuous variables and the chi-square or Fisher's exact test for dichotomous variables. We also compared baseline characteristics for Gr-tol and Gr-intol by the same statistical approach. Multiple logistic regression analysis was used to determine independent predictors of OT and to obtain odds ratios (OR) that were adjusted for possible confounding factors. All the variables found to be different at $P < 0.10$, notably: HLA-A mismatch; early rejection; tacrolimus trough levels within the first week; and time after Tx; as well as those thought to be important on logical and/or biomedical grounds, notably: HLA-B/HLA-DR mismatch, and ABO compatibility, were entered into logistic regression analysis. An early episode of rejection and average tacrolimus trough levels within the first week had been reported to affect OT [29,34]. A trough level of tacrolimus administered orally was adjusted to that administered intravenously (intravenous = per oral × 1.4) [35]. Follow-up (time after Tx) was also included. The 95% confidence interval for each OR was calculated. Statistical significance was determined by 95% confidence intervals not including 1.00 for logistic analyses. Software for this analysis and all other statistical analyses reported here was Stata version 11 (Stata, College Station, TX).

IS protocol

In brief, patients are currently immunosuppressed with tacrolimus and low-dose steroids [16]. As an induction therapy, cyclosporine A was administered with steroids for the first 14 cases, and then it was switched to tacrolimus for all subsequent patients. For the next 60 cases, tacrolimus was continuously given intravenously immediately after LDLT. Subsequently, it was given orally

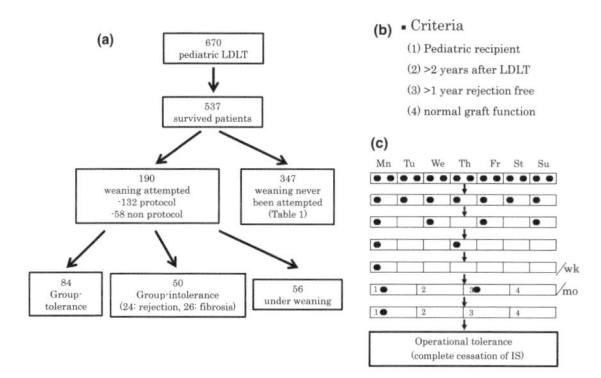

Figure 1 (a) Outcome of Weaning in 670 pediatric patients who underwent LDLT. Of the total number, 537 patients survived. A total of 190 patients attempted weaning immunosuppression (IS) either electively or nonelectively. Eighty four patients successfully discontinued IS, whereas 50 patients were unable to stop IS. Of these, 24 patients failed because of clinically overt rejection after or during the process of weaning IS, whereas 26 patients failed because of fibrosis detected by protocol biopsy. (b) Criteria for selection for the elective weaning protocol. Patients who satisfied the criteria started the Kyoto elective protocol for weaning IS. (c) Protocol for weaning off tacrolimus. The frequency of tacrolimus administration was gradually decreased with intervals of 3–6 months for each step as follows: conventional b.i.d.; q.d.; four times a week; twice a week; once a week; twice a month; once a month, and finally it was completely stopped.

from 1 day pre-Tx for all patients. In our current protocol, the target trough level of tacrolimus was 10–12 ng/ml for the first 2 weeks and 5–10 ng/ml for the following 2 months. After discharge, the dose of tacrolimus was determined individually, depending upon each patient's condition. Steroids were started during LDLT, and were then tapered gradually and stopped after 3 months.

Patients began the weaning protocol when they fulfilled the following criteria [15]: greater than 2 years post-LDLT; normal graft function and no episodes of rejection for more than 1 year (Figure 1). The frequency of tacrolimus administration was reduced in steps (Figure 1). In addition, some patients stopped IS nonelectively mainly because of complications of IS, or noncompliance [15,16]. During the weaning process or after the cessation of IS, patients were carefully monitored for rejection by serum transaminase assay. When an increase in transaminases was observed, the dosage of tacrolimus was increased or corticosteroid pulse therapy was administered with or without assessment of graft histology (deemed intolerance). Additional immunosuppressants such as Orthoclone (OKT3) were used to counteract steroid-resistant rejection [16].

Protocol biopsy

Since January 2003, protocol biopsy of liver grafts has been performed at 1, 2, 5, and 10 years post-Tx on pediatric LDLT patients, even in the presence of a normal liver test. If the biopsy showed pathologic features consistent with acute or chronic rejection, IS was increased and the patients were included in Gr-rej. If advanced fibrosis (bridging fibrosis) was observed by single biopsy, or progression of fibrosis by repeated biopsy, tapering was interrupted and IS was increased [32]. Those cases were included in Gr-fib because fibrosis is regarded as a symptom of rejection, especially as it usually improves after the re-introduction of IS [31].

HLA typing

Haplotypes were serologically defined for HLA-A, HLA-B, and HLA-DR loci in donors and recipients according to the standard methods of the NIH, except emergency LDLT for fulminant hepatitis [36].

Isolation of peripheral blood mononuclear cells

Venous blood was taken from tolerant and intolerant patients who were followed by Kyoto University hospital. Also the venous blood was taken from age-matched healthy volunteers. Peripheral blood mononuclear cells (PBMCs) were isolated from whole blood by density gradient centrifugation over Ficoll-Paque PLUS™ (GE Healthcare Bio-sciences, Uppsala, Sweden). PBMCs were washed twice with phosphate-buffered saline containing

0.1% sodium azide (Wako, Osaka, Japan) and 2% fetal calf serum [18,21].

Fluorescence-activated cell sorting analysis

Cells were stained for 30 min at 4 °C with the following fluorescence-conjugated mAbs: Allophycocyanin-conjugated anti-CD4, PeCy7-conjugated anti-CD25, and phycoerythrin-conjugated anti-IL7-Rα. All mAbs and their isotype controls were purchased from BD Biosciences. The cells were acquired with a FACS Calibur Becton Dickinson Pharmingen (San Diego, CA, USA) and analyzed with BD CellQuest software version 3.3. The frequency of $CD4^+CD25^{++}IL\text{-}7R\alpha^{low+}$ cells was analyzed by the "t"-test. The Human Research Ethics Committee of the Faculty of Medicine, Kyoto University approved this study. Informed consent was provided for pediatric patients according to the Declaration of Helsinki [37].

Results

Outcome of weaning IS

Five-hundred and thirty-seven pediatric patients of 670 patients survived at analysis (April 2008) (Figure 1). Of these, 347 patients had never been assessed as weaning IS, and were excluded from this analysis (Table 1). One-hundred and ninety patients were assessed as weaning IS. Among them, 132 patients were weaned by our elective protocol, and 58 patients stopped IS nonelectively (Figure 1). Eighty-four patients (15.6% of all the surviving patients) were included in Gr-tol (50 electively and 34 nonelectively weaned). Fifty patients were included in Gr-intol (31 electively and 19 nonelectively). Among them, 24 patients encountered acute cellular rejection (Gr-rej) while fibrosis was detected by liver biopsy in 26 patients (Gr-fib). Weaning IS was in progress in 56 patients at the time of this analysis (Figure 1).

Characteristics of excluded patients

Immunosuppression withdrawal had never been attempted in 347 patients, and they remained on maintenance IS (Table 1). Eighty-five of these patients (25%) exhibited unstable liver tests. Ninety-three patients (27%) had not been followed up at Kyoto University Hospital and their current clinical status and laboratory data were missing. In 18 patients (8%), although liver function was stable, weaning IS had never been attempted because of the absence of collaboration of local physicians. The other patients did not satisfy the criteria because of the presence of fibrosis or insufficient time from Tx (<2 years) (Table 1).

Table 1. Characteristics of excluded patients.

	Excluded patients (n = 347)	Patients not followed up (n = 93)
Recipient age in years, mean (SD)	5.2 (5.1)	5.4 (5.1)
Recipient female, N (%)	214 (63%)	61 (66%)
Underlying disease, N (%)		
Biliary atresia	256 (76%)	68 (73%)
Blood test before Tx, mean (SD)		
WBC (X10³/l)	7.9 (5.4)	7.7 (5.0)
PLT (X10³/μl)	185.5 (309.2)	229.5 (549.2)
CRP (mg/dl)	1.6 (2.8)	1.8 (3.6)
AST (U/l)	191 (156)	180 (129)
ALT (U/l)	128 (141)	108 (90)
Albumin (mg/dl)	3.6 (0.6)	3.6 (0.6)
Total bilirubin (mg/dl)	11.6 (10.3)	11.6 (10.0)
Creatinine (mg/dl)	0.28 (0.23)	0.29 (0.23)
PT (s)	15.0 (5.5)	14.7 (4.9)
Condition, N (%)		
Hospitalized	207 (62%)	54 (58%)
Donor age in years, mean (SD)	35.3 (7.9)	34.7 (8.0)
Donor female, N (%)	172 (51%)	49 (53%)
ABO compatible, N (%)	287 (84%)	81 (87%)
Graft weight (GRBW%), mean (SD)	2.3 (1.1)	2.3 (1.2)
Follow up time after Tx in days, mean (SD)	2787 (1492)	3629 (1151)
The reason for not weaning, N (%)		
unstable LFT	85 (25%)	
ACR	45 (13%)	
fibrosis	19 (6%)	
AIH	16 (5%)	
CR	12 (4%)	
APOLT	3 (1%)	
re-Transplantation	16 (5%)	
not followed up	93 (27%)	
stable, but not assessed as weaning	18 (8%)	
other	5 (1%)	
<2 years after transplantation	37 (11%)	

LFT, liver function test; ACR, acute cellular rejection; AIH, autoimmune hepatitis; CR, chronic rejection; APOLT, auxiliary partial orthotopic liver transplantation. WBC, white blood cell; PLT, platelet; CRP, C-reactive protein; AST, aspartate aminotransferase; ALT, alanine aminotransferase; PT, prothrombin time; GRBW, graft recipient to body weight.

Characteristics of eligible patients

Fifty patients who were not able to fulfill the requirement for OT were included, consisting of patients who had acute or chronic rejection (Gr-rej), and those who had advanced or progressive fibrosis (Gr-fib). The characteristics of Gr-rej and Gr-fib patients are compared in Table 2. There was a significant difference between the groups ($P < 0.001$) in the reason for IS withdrawal as Gr-rej had been mainly nonelectively

Table 2. Characteristics of Gr-rej and Gr-fib patients.

	Group-rejection (n = 24)	Group-fibrosis (n = 26)	P value
Recipient age in years, mean (SD)	2.0 (3.3)	2.2 (2.6)	0.9
Recipient female, N (%)	18 (75%)	18 (69%)	0.7
Underlying disease, N (%)			
Biliary atresia	21 (88%)	22 (85%)	0.8
Blood test before transplantation, mean (SD)			
WBC (×10^3/l)	8.6 (4.0)	8.0 (5.7)	0.7
PLT (×10^3/μl)	161.6 (77.3)	153.1 (86.0)	0.7
CRP (mg/dl)	1.5 (1.4)	3.2 (4.8)	0.1
AST (U/l)	270 (157)	223 (136)	0.3
ALT (U/l)	143 (81)	145 (108)	0.9
Albumin (mg/dl)	3.5 (0.6)	3.5 (0.7)	1.0
Total bilirubin (mg/dl)	13.2 (12.4)	15.4 (10.0)	0.5
Creatinine (mg/dl)	0.18 (0.08)	0.15 (0.05)	0.2
PT (s)	14.9 (5.6)	15.8 (6.3)	0.6
Condition, N (%)			
Hospitalized	12 (50%)	15 (58%)	0.6
Donor age in years, mean (SD)	31.8 (8.3)	31.0 (4.3)	0.7
ABO compatible, N (%)	18 (75%)	25 (96%)	0.03
Graft weight (GRBW%), mean (SD)	3.2 (1.2)	3.0 (1.0)	0.9
The presence of HLA-A mismatch, N (%)	17 (85%)	23 (92%)	0.5
The presence of HLA-B mismatch, N (%)	17 (85%)	23 (92%)	0.5
The presence of HLA-DR mismatch, N (%)	16 (80%)	22 (88%)	0.5
The absence of early rejection, N (%)	13 (54%)	17 (65%)	0.4
Tacrolimus level (ng/ml), mean (SD) (average within the first week post-LDLT) all adjusted to intravenous level	14.8 (5.9)	14.9 (4.3)	1.0
Reason for IS withdrawal			<0.001
Protocol, N (%)	7 (29%)	24 (92%)	
Infection, N (%)	14 (58%)	1 (4%)	
Others, N (%)	3 (13%)	1 (4%)	
Follow-up time after Tx in days, mean (SD)	3889 (1236)	4418 (906)	0.08

HLA, human leukocyte antigen; LDLT, living-donor liver transplants; IS, immunosuppression.

weaned because of infection whereas Gr-fib were almost all weaned according to protocol. The only other difference was a higher incidence of ABO compatibility in Gr-fib (96%) compared with Gr-rej (75%) (P = 0.03). Other factors of clinical significance between the groups, such as HLA mismatch and absence of early rejection were quite similar and because of this they were pooled (Gr-intol) for univariate and multivariate analysis.

Univariate analysis of Gr-tol and Gr-intol is shown in Table 3. Patients in Gr-intol had experienced rejection within the first month post-LDLT at a significantly higher incidence (40%) than Gr-tol (17%) (P < 0.01). The average trough level of tacrolimus within the first week post-LDLT was significantly higher in Gr-tol (17.1 ng/ml) than in Gr-intol (11.0 ng/ml) (P < 0.01). In addition, the follow-up time (time after Tx) in Gr-tol (4 725 days) was significantly longer than Gr-intol (4 135 days) (P < 0.01). No other parameters differed between the two, although a higher rate of HLA-A mismatch in Gr-intol approached significance (P = 0.07).

Multivariate analysis of Gr-tol versus Gr-intol

Multivariate analysis is shown in Table 4. The absence of early rejection was associated with OT and had an OR (95% CI) of 2.79 (1.11–7.02) (P = 0.03). Matching at the HLA-A locus was also associated with OT with an OR of 0.18 (0.03–0.91) (P = 0.04). ABO compatibility or HLA-DR mismatch was not statistically significant. Higher trough levels of tacrolimus in the first week after Tx showed an association with OT (P = 0.02). In contrast, patients who were matched at the HLA-B locus were less likely to develop tolerance. The OR for HLA-B mismatch was 8.73 (1.09–70.0) (P = 0.04). Although this level is statistically significant, the large confidence interval and the very small percentage of patients in both groups who were matched at HLA-B question its clinical significance.

Factors relevant to tolerance after semi-allogeneic liver transplantation   Ohe et al.

Table 3. Univariate analysis of Gr-tol versus Gr-intol patients.

	Group-tolerance (n = 84)	Group-intolerance (n = 50)	P value
Recipient age in years, mean (SD)	2.9 (3.7)	2.1 (2.9)	0.20
Recipient female, N (%)	49 (58%)	36 (72%)	0.11
Underlying disease, N (%)			
Biliary atresia	67 (80%)	43 (86%)	0.36
Blood test before transplantation, mean (SD)			
WBC (X10^3/l)	8.0 (4.6)	8.3 (5.0)	0.78
PLT (X10^3/μl)	169.7 (101.8)	157.2 (81.2)	0.46
CRP (mg/dl)	2.1 (2.4)	2.4 (3.7)	0.63
AST (U/l)	235 (157.8)	245 (147.1)	0.70
ALT (U/l)	134 (103.2)	144 (94.8)	0.58
Albumin (mg/dl)	3.5 (0.7)	3.5 (0.6)	0.59
Total bilirubin (mg/dl)	15.8 (9.5)	14.3 (11.1)	0.41
Creatinine (mg/dl)	0.18 (0.08)	0.16 (0.07)	0.28
PT (s)	14.3 (3.2)	15.4 (5.9)	0.21
Condition, N (%)			
Hospitalized	51 (61%)	30 (60%)	0.87
Donor age in years, mean (SD)	33.0 (6.3)	31.4 (6.5)	0.15
ABO compatible, N (%)	77 (92%)	43 (86%)	0.30
Graft weight (GRBW%), mean (SD)	2.9 (1.3)	3.1 (1.1)	0.32
The presence of HLA-A mismatch, N (%)	54 (75%)	40 (89%)	0.07
The presence of HLA-B mismatch, N (%)	68 (94%)	40 (89%)	0.27
The presence of HLA-DR mismatch, N (%)	60 (83%)	38 (84%)	0.87
The absence of early rejection, N (%)	70 (83%)	30 (60%)	<0.01
Tacrolimus trough level (ng/ml), mean (SD) (average within the first week post-LDLT)	17.1 (12.0)	11.0 (5.1)	<0.01
Reason for IS withdrawal			0.2
Protocol, N (%)	50 (60%)	31 (62%)	
Infection, N (%)	18 (22%)	15 (30%)	
Others, N (%)	15 (18%)	4 (8%)	
Follow up time after Tx in days, mean (SD)	4725 (1102.3)	4135 (1098.9)	<0.01

HLA, human leukocyte antigen; LDLT, living-donor liver transplants; IS, immunosuppression.

Table 4. Multivariate analysis of Gr-tol versus Gr-intol.

Variable	P value	Odds ratio	95% CI
ABO compatible	0.720	1.41	0.22–8.94
The absence of early rejection	0.030	2.79	1.11–7.02
The presence of HLA-A mismatch	0.040	0.18	0.03–0.91
The presence of HLA-B mismatch	0.040	8.73	1.09–70.0
The presence of HLA-DR mismatch	0.710	0.78	0.21–2.84
Follow up time after Tx (days)	0.22	1	1.00–1.00
Tacrolimus trough level	0.020	1.104	1.016–1.200

HLA, human leukocyte antigen; CI, confidence interval.

Frequency of CD4$^+$CD25^{++}IL-7Rα^{low+} cells

Blood samples could be obtained from 32 of 134 patients enrolled in this study. Of them, 24 patients were Gr-tol whereas eight were in Gr-intol. The frequency of CD4$^+$CD25^{++}IL-7Rα^{low+} cells within the peripheral CD4$^+$ cells at more than 10 years post-Tx was significantly decreased in the Gr-intol cohort (4.9 ± 1.0%) compared with the Gr-tol cohort (7.6 ± 1.7%) (P = 0.003) (Figure 2a). Twenty-five patients were HLA-A mismatched whereas seven were matched. The HLA-A mismatched cohort included 19 tolerant and 6 intolerant patients. The HLA-A matched cohort included five tolerant and two intolerant patients. The frequency of CD4$^+$CD25^{++}IL-7Rα^{low+} cells was comparable between the HLA-A matched cohort and the mismatched cohort (7.2 ± 2.6 vs. 6.9 ± 1.8%, HLA-A matched vs. mismatch, P = 0.761) (Figure 2b). In contrast, there were fewer CD4$^+$CD25^{++}IL-7Rα^{low+} cells in the HLA-B matched cohort compared with the HLA-B mismatched cohort and healthy volunteers (4.7 ± 1.1 vs. 7.3 ± 1.9, 9.0 ± 2.9%, HLA-B matched vs. mismatch, P = 0.011, HLA-B match vs. healthy volunteers, P = 0.013) (Figure 2c), although the low numbers in the matched cohort question the validity of this result.

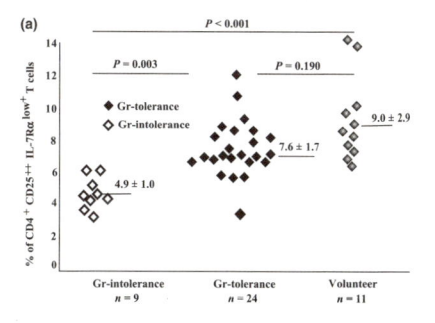

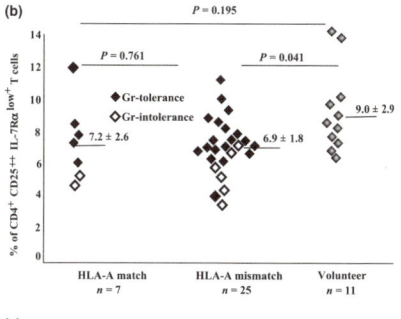

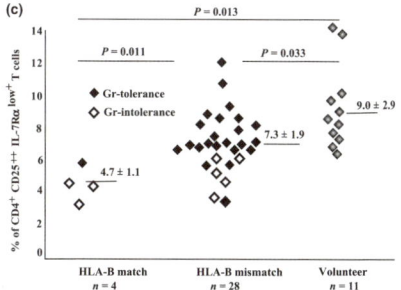

Figure 2 The frequency of CD4⁺CD25⁺⁺IL-7Rα^low+ T cells with HLA match. (a) The frequency of CD4⁺CD25⁺⁺IL-7Rα^low+ T cells between group-tolerance versus group-intolerance. Of 134 patients, peripheral blood was available for phenotypic analyses in 33 patients. The frequency of CD4⁺CD25⁺⁺IL-7Rα^low+ T cells within CD4⁺ cells was significantly lower in Gr-intol than that in Gr-tol (at >10 years post-Tx) (4.9 ± 1.0 vs. 7.6 ± 1.7%, Gr-intol vs. Gr-tol, $P = 0.003$). (b) Effect of HLA-A match. The frequency of CD4⁺CD25⁺⁺IL-7Rα^low+ T cells within CD4⁺ cells did not differ between the HLA-A matched and mismatched cohorts (7.2 ± 2.6 vs. 6.9 ± 1.8%, HLA-A matched vs. mismatched, $P = 0.761$). (c) Effect of HLA-B match. In the HLA-B matched cohort, the frequency of CD4⁺CD25⁺⁺IL-7Rα^low+ T cells within CD4⁺ cells was significantly decreased compared with those in the HLA-B mismatch cohort and age-matched healthy volunteers (4.7 ± 1.1 vs. 7.3 ± 1.9, 9.0 ± 2.9%, HLA-B matched vs. mismatched, $P = 0.011$, HLA-B match vs. healthy volunteers, $P = 0.013$).

reported that advanced fibrosis or progression of fibrosis is an indicator of the need for increased IS, we compared patients who required recommencement of IS because of rejection with those who had IS restarted for fibrosis. Characteristics for these two groups were similar; with the notable exception of the reason for IS withdrawal, where the majority of the patients in Gr-rej had been rapidly weaned nonelectively mainly due to Epstein-Barr virus infection [16] whereas Gr-fib patients were almost all electively weaned according to protocol. Perhaps, the rapid removal of the Gr-rej patients from IS during nonelective weaning predisposes these patients to frank rejection that is easily diagnosed on the basis of graft pathology on biopsy. In contrast, the slower removal of IS according to protocol of the Gr-fib patients might have led to a low-grade immune response to the graft that manifests itself as graft fibrosis in these patients. This is especially the case as long-term pediatric liver transplant recipients show a very high tendency to develop fibrosis in association with inflammation [38]. An alternative explanation is that severe viral infection could induce cross-reactive (heterologous) immunity that increases the likelihood of rejection, as shown in animal models [39]. Further statistical analysis of the two separate intolerant groups could not be performed, because of their small sample sizes. However, it will be interesting to compare other immune parameters such as extent and type of antibody deposited, composition of cellular infiltrate, and expression of cytokines and growth factors.

As both the intolerant groups were similar in other clinical features, except for the incidence of ABO compatibility, which was higher in the fibrosis group, they were combined for further analysis (Gr-intol). Comparison of Gr-tol with Gr-intol showed that the presence of rejection episodes in the first month was associated with intolerance, which accords well with published findings [29].

Discussion

This is the first retrospective analysis of weaning of IS in a large cohort of living-related (parent to child) pediatric liver Tx patients. Although parent to child (F1) Tx are not as common as deceased donor Tx, the lack of sufficient deceased donors has led to their increasing incidence in both liver and kidney Tx. As we have previously

Increased levels of trough tacrolimus in the first week after Tx have been associated with OT of liver Tx patients, which is supported by the findings reported here. Although HLA matching is not thought to play a role in the outcome of deceased donor liver Tx, we found that matching at the HLA-A locus was associated with OT in this pediatric LDLT population, which is in accordance with the findings of improved outcomes in HLA-A matched patients in deceased donor renal Tx [22–25].

In contrast to these published results, we describe here a statistically significant association between HLA-B mismatch and OT in the multivariate, but not the univariate analysis. This finding is unexpected as in the setting of renal Tx, mismatches of HLA-B between donors and recipients negatively impact the outcomes of graft survival more strongly than those of other HLA loci [40]. This is in accordance with the *in vitro* observations that HLA-B is more immunogenic than HLA-A and HLA-DR [41]. Therefore, our findings in LDLT patients stand in contrast to those in both liver and kidney Tx patients. Consequently, it is tempting to discount this effect as a statistical aberration, because of the very small proportion of HLA-B matched patients in both groups with a consequent large confidence interval and the lack of significance in the univariate analysis. Despite this, some support for the finding comes from the completely independent area of maternal/fetal tolerance. In the Hutterites (an inbred population of European descent), significantly increased fetal loss rates were observed among couples matched for HLA-B [42]. Thus, if our findings that HLA-B mismatch favorably affects OT are correct, they appear to be consistent with maternal/fetal tolerance, suggesting that there may be common features between the two.

Recently, we have shown that donor-antigen specific regulatory T cells (Tregs) can be generated in LDLT patients and play a critical role in the induction and the maintenance of OT [18–21]. Our data are consistent with those in deceased liver Tx and kidney Tx reported by others [43,44]. The findings here in an expanded population confirm that the frequency of $CD4^+CD25^{++}IL-7R\alpha^{low+}$ Tregs within the peripheral $CD4^+$ cells derived from Gr-intol patients were significantly decreased compared with Gr-tol patients. Of interest, there was a higher percentage of Tregs in the HLA-B-mismatched patients which is in agreement with our findings of an improved outcome in HLA-B mismatched recipients. Such a correlation was not observed between HLA-A and Tregs, despite the association between HLA-A matching and tolerance. However, there are very small numbers of patients in the mismatched groups which questions the validity of these results.

Some potential limitations of the present study should be considered. Firstly, a large number of patients in the original cohort were excluded because they were not being followed up or had not been assessed as weaning. However, examination of the baseline characteristics of those patients showed that they were similar to those included in the study, suggesting that selection bias was not a major issue. Second, it is unclear whether the results reported here for HLA matching and OT in semi-allogeneic pediatric LDLT can be generalized to fully allogeneic deceased donor liver Tx. The original studies of MHC restriction by Zinkernagel and Doherty showed that F1 targets behaved similar to fully allogeneic targets [45]. Similarly, in NK cell-mediated killing of target cells lacking MHC expression, first described by Karre, there was a quantitative, but not a qualitative difference between F1 and fully allogeneic systems [46]. In animal models of liver Tx tolerance and rejection, there was also a quantitative rather than a qualitative difference between F1 and fully allogeneic grafts, with the F1 showing an outcome that was intermediate between the two parental strains [47]. On the basis of these findings, results here may be extended, to some degree, to fully allogeneic grafts.

A third factor that could influence the outcome was that this study included patients who started weaning IS electively and stopped nonelectively. It is possible that this could lead to heterogeneity of patients that could jeopardize analyses. However, regardless of weaning being elective or nonelective, the probability of successful cessation of IS was comparable between Gr-Tol or Gr-Intol (Table 3). The main difference we observed between elective and nonelective weaning was its effect on rejection compared to fibrosis as a cause of intolerance as discussed above. It is also possible that subjects enrolled in this study could have been heterogeneous in terms of IS administration as this was changed over the course of the study. Initially, IS was delivered intravenously and later orally. To adjust for this, the trough level of tacrolimus administered orally was multiplied by 1.4, according to a published report [35]. Finally, the possibility that surgical techniques and post-Tx management were modified with time was taken into account.

In conclusion, this is the first retrospective analysis from a large cohort of pediatric LDLT patients examining factors which affect the subsequent development of tolerance. This is the first demonstration that HLA-A matching may be one of the determinants for OT in semi-allogeneic pediatric liver transplantation. It accords with the previously reported association between tolerance and absence of early rejection episodes in deceased donor recipients of liver Tx. The association between higher levels of Tregs in tolerant patients is consistent with previous studies [18–21,43,44]. Last but not least, we cannot rule out the possibility that both rejection and fibrosis play a different role in the pathologic progression of intolerance. Further large scale studies are needed to identify clinically significant effects of differences between rejection and fibrosis that lead to post-Tx intolerance.

Authorship

HO, KW, MY, HN-H, YL, XZ, TM and TK: carried out the research. HO, HN-H, YL, TK, SS and AB: wrote the manuscript. TK: participated in research design. HO, KW and HN-H: conducted the data analysis. SU: directed the transplant program.

Funding

This work was supported by the Ministry of Education, Culture, Sports, Science and Technology of Japan as well as Astellas Pharma Inc. Tokyo.

Acknowledgements

We thank Prof. J Pirenne, Prof. KJ Wood, Dr. A Nakao, Dr. T Toyosaki-Maeda, Dr. H Saji, Prof. M Fukushima Dr. E Ogura, and Prof. A Shintani for helpful discussions and the critical reading of this manuscript, and Dr. JD Parker for manuscript preparation.

References

1. Ueda M, Oike F, Ogura Y, *et al.* Long-term outcomes of 600 living donor liver transplants for pediatric patients at a single center. *Liver Transpl* 2006; **12**: 1326.
2. Jonas S, Neuhaus R, Junge G, *et al.* Primary immunosuppression with tacrolimus after liver transplantation: 12-years follow-up. *Int Immunopharmacol* 2005; **5**: 125.
3. Matthews J, Ramos E, Bluestone J. Clinical trials of transplant tolerance: slow but steady progress. *Am J Transplant* 2003; **3**: 794.
4. Tisone G, Orlando G, Angelico M. Operational tolerance in clinical liver transplantation: emerging developments. *Transpl Immunol* 2007; **17**: 108.
5. Roussey-Kesler G, Giral M, Moreau A, *et al.* Clinical operational tolerance after kidney transplantation. *Am J Transplant* 2006; **6**: 736.
6. Auchincloss HJ. In search of the elusive Holy Grail: the mechanisms and prospects for achieving clinical transplantation tolerance. *Am J Transplant* 2001; **1**: 6.
7. Cuturi M, Josien R, Douillard P, *et al.* Prolongation of allogeneic heart graft survival in rats by administration of a peptide (a.a. 75–84) from the alpha 1 helix of the first domain of HLA-B7 01. *Transplantation* 1995; **59**: 661.
8. Gianello P, Fishbein J, Sachs D. Tolerance to primarily vascularized allografts in miniature swine. *Immunol Rev* 1993; **133**: 19.
9. Knechtle S. Knowledge about transplantation tolerance gained in primates. *Curr Opin Immunol* 2000; **12**: 552.
10. Levisetti M, Padril P, Szot G, *et al.* Immunosuppressive effects of human CTLA4Ig in a non-human primate model of allogeneic pancreatic islet transplantation. *J Immunol* 1997; **159**: 5187.
11. Remuzzi G, Rossini M, Imberti O, Perico N. Kidney graft survival in rats without immunosuppressants after intrathymic glomerular transplantation. *Lancet* 1991; **337**: 750.
12. Sablinski T, Hancock W, Tilney N, Kupiec-Weglinski J. CD4 monoclonal antibodies in organ transplantation – a review of progress. *Transplantation* 1991; **52**: 579.
13. Subbotin V, Sun H, Aitouche A, *et al.* Abrogation of chronic rejection in a murine model of aortic allotransplantation by prior induction of donor-specific tolerance. *Transplantation* 1997; **64**: 690.
14. Starzl T, Demetris A, Trucco M, *et al.* Chimerism and donor-specific nonreactivity 27 to 29 years after kidney allotransplantation. *Transplantation* 1993; **55**: 1272.
15. Takatsuki M, Uemoto S, Inomata Y, *et al.* Weaning of immunosuppression in living donor liver transplant recipients. *Transplantation* 2001; **72**: 449.
16. Koshiba T, Li Y, Takemura M, *et al.* Clinical, immunological, and pathological aspects of operational tolerance after pediatric living-donor liver transplantation. *Transpl Immunol* 2007; **17**: 94.
17. Cortesini R. Tolerance in clinical liver transplantation. *Transpl Immunol* 2007; **17**: 81.
18. Li Y, Koshiba T, Yoshizawa A, *et al.* Analyses of peripheral blood mononuclear cells in operational tolerance after pediatric living donor liver transplantation. *Am J Transplant* 2004; **4**: 2118.
19. Li Y, Zhao X, Cheng D, *et al.* The presence of Foxp3 expressing T cells within grafts of tolerant human liver transplant recipients. *Transplantation* 2008; **86**: 1837.
20. Yoshizawa A, Ito A, Li Y, *et al.* The roles of CD25+CD4+ regulatory T cells in operational tolerance after living donor liver transplantation. *Transplant Proc* 2005; **37**: 37.
21. Nafady-Hego H, Li Y, Ohe H, *et al.* The generation of donor-specific CD4+CD25++CD45RA+ naive regulatory T cells in operationally tolerant patients after pediatric living-donor liver transplantation. *Transplantation* 2010; **90**: 1547.
22. Dausset J, Hors J, Busson M, *et al.* Serologically defined HL-A antigens and long-term survival of cadaver kidney transplants. A joint analysis of 918 cases performed by France-Transplant and the London Transplant Group. *N Engl J Med* 1974; **290**: 979.
23. Persijn G, Cohen B, Lansbergen Q, *et al.* Effect of HLA-A and HLA-B matching on survival of grafts and recipients after renal transplantation. *N Engl J Med* 1982; **307**: 905.
24. Opelz G. Importance of HLA antigen splits for kidney transplant matching. *Lancet* 1988; **2**: 61.
25. Opelz G. The benefit of exchanging donor kidneys among transplant centers. *N Engl J Med* 1988; **318**: 1289.
26. Neumann U, Guckelberger O, Langrehr J, *et al.* Impact of human leukocyte antigen matching in liver transplantation. *Transplantation* 2003; **75**: 132.

27. Navarro V, Herrine S, Katopes C, Colombe B, Spain C. The effect of HLA class I (A and B) and class II (DR) compatibility on liver transplantation outcomes: an analysis of the OPTN database. *Liver Transpl* 2006; **12**: 652.
28. Sieders E, Hepkema B, Peeters P, *et al*. The effect of HLA mismatches, shared cross-reactive antigen groups, and shared HLA-DR antigens on the outcome after pediatric liver transplantation. *Liver Transpl* 2005; **11**: 1541.
29. Devlin J, Doherty D, Thomson L, *et al*. Defining the outcome of immunosuppression withdrawal after liver transplantation. *Hepatology* 1998; **27**: 926.
30. Tryphonopoulos P, Ruiz P, Weppler D, *et al*. Long-term follow-up of 23 operational tolerant liver transplant recipients. *Transplantation* 2010; **90**: 1536.
31. Ohe H, Li Y, Nafady-Hego H, *et al*. Minimal but essential doses of immunosuppression: a more realistic approach to improve long-term outcomes for pediatric living-donor liver transplantation. *Transplantation* 2011; **91**: 808.
32. Yoshitomi M, Koshiba T, Haga H, *et al*. Requirement of protocol biopsy before and after complete cessation of immunosuppression after liver transplantation. *Transplantation* 2009; **87**: 606.
33. Tanaka K, Uemoto S, Tokunaga Y, *et al*. Surgical techniques and innovations in living related liver transplantation. *Ann Surg* 1993; **217**: 82.
34. Tisone G, Orlando G, Cardillo A, *et al*. Complete weaning off immunosuppression in HCV liver transplant recipients is feasible and favourably impacts on the progression of disease recurrence. *J Hepatol* 2006; **44**: 702.
35. Undre N, Moller A. Pharmacokinetic interpretation of FK 506 levels in blood and in plasma during a European randomised study in primary liver transplant patients. The FK 506 European Study Group. *Transplant Int* 1994; **7**(Suppl 1): S15.
36. Kasahara M, Kiuchi T, Uryuhara K, *et al*. Role of HLA compatibility in pediatric living-related liver transplantation. *Transplantation* 2002; **74**: 1175.
37. Burns JP. Research in children. *Crit Care Med* 2003; **31**(3 Suppl): S131.
38. Ekong UD, Melin-Aldana H, Seshadri R, *et al*. Graft histology characteristics in long-term survivors of pediatric liver transplantation. *Liver Transplant* 2008; **14**: 1582.
39. Adams AB, Williams MA, Jones TR, *et al*. Heterologous immunity provides a potent barrier to transplantation tolerance. *J Clin Invest* 2003; **111**: 1887.
40. Roelen DL, van Bree SP, van Beelen E, Schanz U, van Rood JJ, Claas FH. Cytotoxic T lymphocytes against HLA-B antigens are less naive than cytotoxic T lymphocytes against HLA-A antigens. *Transplantation* 1994; **57**: 446.
41. Zhang L, van Bree S, van Rood JJ, Claas FH. The effect of individual HLA-A and -B mismatches on the generation of cytotoxic T lymphocyte precursors. *Transplantation* 1990; **50**: 1008.
42. Ober C, Hyslop T, Elias S, Weitkamp L, Hauck W. Human leukocyte antigen matching and fetal loss: results of a 10 year prospective study. *Hum Reprod* 1998; **13**: 33.
43. Martínez-Llordella M, Puig-Pey I, Orlando G, *et al*. Multiparameter immune profiling of operational tolerance in liver transplantation. *Am J Transplant* 2007; **7**: 309.
44. Louis S, Braudeau C, Giral M, *et al*. Contrasting CD25hiCD4+T cells/FOXP3 patterns in chronic rejection and operational drug-free tolerance. *Transplantation* 2006; **81**: 398.
45. Zinkernagel RM, Doherty PC. H-2 compatibility requirement for T-cell-mediated lysis of target cells infected with lymphocytic choriomeningitis virus. Different cytotoxic T-cell specificities are associated with structures coded for in H-2K or H-2D. *J Exp Med* 1975; **141**: 1427.
46. Karre K, Ljunggren HG, Piontek G, Kiessling R. Selective rejection of H-2-deficient lymphoma variants suggests alternative immune defence strategy. *Nature* 1986; **319**: 675.
47. Kamada N. The immunology of experimental liver transplantation in the rat. *Immunology* 1985; **55**: 369.

（Ohe H, et al.：Factors affecting operational tolerance after pediatric living-donor liver transplantation: impact of early post-transplant events and HLA match. *Transpl Int* 2012;25:97-106. 許諾を得て転載）

まとめ

「はじめに」でも述べた循環器領域で全世界で最も有名で最もよく読まれている論文誌 JACC の DeMaria 編集長からの，論文執筆アドバイスの 10 点に筆者の解釈を加えたのが以下である．

① 研究の仮説がある（はず）
　観察研究であっても，病態や仮説生成に結びつける仮説がある．
② 「新しさ」を記載
　過去の知見の確認や別のセッティングでの一般化可能性も「新しさ」である．
③ Methods は詳細に
　患者採用手法や研究群（含：対照群）の適切さ，アウトカムや変数評価の公平性が重要である．
④ サンプルサイズ計算
　RCT では必須である．
⑤ 一つにまとめるべき研究を切り分けない
　いくつもサブグループ解析論文を不明確な理由で執筆するのではなく，一つのサブグループ解析にもきちんとした理由づけが必要である．
⑥ 丁寧な解析
　1. 原因−結果の因果関係を見ているのか，単に関連性を見ているのか．
　2. エンドポイントは surrogate なのか真の outcome なのか．
　3. 交絡因子はきちんと考慮されているか．
⑦ Results についてきちんと Discussion で考察
　第 1 パラグラフで主要な Results をまとめる．
⑧ Table と Figure の重要性
　一目瞭然の Table と Figure を作成する．
⑨ 論文全体のバランス
　1. Title から最後の Reference，図表までの質感のよさ，バランスが重要である．
　2. 極端な話，著者数 ＞ 患者数という論文はどうなのか？
　3. Results に比して Conclusion の分量が多い論文は，針小棒大？
⑩ 無駄な努力
　cover letter でやたら研究の重要性を強調したところで，わかる人はわかる．

まとめ

JACC Editors の 10 のアドバイス

① 研究の仮説がある（はず）	⑥ 丁寧な解析
②「新しさ」を記載	⑦ Results についてきちんと Discussion で考察
③ Methods は詳細に	⑧ Table と Figure の重要性
④ サンプルサイズ計算	⑨ 論文全体のバランス
⑤ 一つにまとめるべき研究を切り分けない	⑩ 無駄な努力

(DeMaria AN：How do I get a paper accepted?–Part 2. J Am Coll Cardiol 2007；49：1989-90)

　最後に，本書のまとめとして，筆者が考えるよい論文を書くためのポイントを列挙したい．

① 読者，査読者，編集者が読みやすい論文
　RCT なら RCT，横断研究なら横断研究の論文に必要な要素は決まっていて，それが論旨に矛盾なくすっと入ってくるか？　共著者が何人もいるにも関わらず，読みにくいのは，ほぼ間違いなく共著者が論文のドラフトに関わっていない証拠である．共著者がちゃんと読めば，読みにくいものは読みにくいと気づくはずである．

② 短い，パラレル構造，一致
　短く書けるものは短く書くほうが，読みやすさにもつながるし，編集者もページの節約ができる．パラレル構造や一致も，引っかかりなく読む重要な要素である．特に論文を推敲する段階では，パラレル構造と一致を確認してほしい．

③ Tables & Figures を有効に使う
　論文誌の投稿規定の最大数まで Tables と Figures を活用し，パッと見てわかる論文に．

④ 対象患者が容易にイメージ
　Methods の記載や Study Flowchart，Table 1 で，どのような患者を対象に研究を行ったのかが，すぐにわかるように．対象患者＝この論文の応用対象であり，論文の社会的インパクトが規定される．

⑤ 再現性のある Methods
　臨床研究はサイエンスである．再現性のない研究はサイエンスではない．特に，統計解析などでは，同じデータがあれば同じ結果が出るようにロジックが明確

な解析手法を使う.

⑥ 研究結果と引用と妄想を区別
Discussion では研究の直接的な観察結果をもとに考察を展開する．他の研究者からの引用と，研究者の思い（妄想）が中心とならないように気をつける．

⑦ 多くの目で書き直し
2回目の自分の目，3回目の自分の目，共著者の目……と多くの目で書き直すことで，編集者や査読者といった「赤の他人」が読むに堪える文章が完成する．もちろん，ロジックの不備も見つかり，早い段階で修正が可能となる．

⑧ 臨床疫学・統計専門家は執筆でも
臨床疫学や統計の専門家は臨床研究のデザインや統計解析で力を発揮するが，論文執筆の際においても，ロジックの整合性や論文全体の consistency などを確認するには頼りになる共著者である．

森本剛からの8つのアドバイス

① 読者，審査員，編集者が読みやすい論文	⑤ 再現性のある Methods
② 短い，パラレル構造，一致	⑥ 研究結果と引用と妄想を区別
③ Tables & Figures を有効に使う	⑦ 多くの目で書き直し
④ 対象患者が容易にイメージ	⑧ 臨床疫学・統計専門家は執筆でも

おわりに

　最近，臨床研究論文の書き方，academic writing の講演依頼が多い．確かに，わが国では研究論文を書くべき若手研究者や医師向けのきちんとした academic writing の教育機会が極端に少ない．筆者自身がきちんとした教育を受けたのか，人にきちんと教育できているかどうか，極めて心許ない．しかしながら，これだけ講演依頼を受けるとそれなりにニーズがあるのではないか，と思う．もちろん，講義だけではダメであり，きちんとした臨床研究を実施し，自分で論文を書くという実践が必要なことは言うまでもないが，少なくともその取りかかりとなる最低限度の基礎教育は必要であろう．本書がその最低限度の教育機会になれば幸いである．これで講演依頼も減ると思うとやれやれである．筆者は講演よりも，もっとわくわくするような臨床研究や若手研究者の研究指導，論文執筆をやりたいのである．

　ちょうどこの原稿を執筆している際に，iPS 細胞臨床応用の捏造・誤報問題が発生した．この問題についてコメントを求められた iPS 細胞の生みの親である山中伸弥教授は「論文を読んでいないので何とも言えない」と答えたと，新聞に報道されていた．これがサイエンスである．学会発表や速報をいくら重ねても，きちんとしたピアレビューを経た学術誌に掲載されなければ，研究そのものの信頼性はないのである．最初の前提でも書いたが，論文を書いて学術誌に報告しなければ，それは研究ではない．研究に関わるすべての研究者は，論文発表という最終成果物までのプロセスを意識して研究に望んでほしい．本書はその道筋のガイドでもある．

　でき上がったドラフトを見ると，総論の第Ⅰ部は意外に分量が少なく，第Ⅱ部が大部分を占めていた．普段の臨床研究教育でも，総論の講義よりも，各論にあたる個別の研究内容についてのディスカッションを多くしているのと同じ傾向になっていた．技能の教育には実務研修が重要なのである．

＊　　＊　　＊

　本書を執筆するにあたって，多くの先生方のお世話になりました．「第Ⅱ部　論文 Before & After」で，快く論文執筆段階初期のドラフトを提供してくださった，作間未織先生，岡田定規先生，塩見紘樹先生，阿部充先生，大江秀典先生に深謝申し上げます．また，筆者に論文執筆のノウハウを直接ご指導くださったのはハーバード大学の David W Bates 先生，Thomas H Lee 先生です．このノウハウをも

とに，たくさんの臨床研究の指導や執筆の機会を与えてくださったのは小川久雄先生，斎藤能彦先生，木村剛先生，植田真一郎先生であり，先生方との実践がなければ本書の内容はありませんでした．

　筆者自身は総合内科医をベースにどんな医学領域の研究にも対応できる academic generalist を目指していますが，筆者に academic generalist への道をご教示いただいた福井次矢先生，松村理司先生，酒見英太先生，松井邦彦先生には，いまだにたくさんのご指導をいただいています．

　最後になりますが，筆者は臨床研究に関わる時間をできるだけ確保するため，ずっと日本語の総説論文や日本語書籍の執筆をお断りしております．本書の執筆も，いつも通り拒む筆者にしつこく執筆のお誘いをいただき，完成までずっとご支援いただいた，中山書店企画室の北原裕一さんに深謝とお恨みを申し上げて，Word® の×をクリックしたいと思います．

平成 24 年 11 月　42 歳の誕生日に
秋深まる京都で

索　引

あ行

引用 ································ 37
英語の掟 ···························· 45
エンドポイント ···················· 28

か行

解析結果 ···························· 28
解析方法 ···························· 25
学会発表 ······························ 8
キーワード ························· 32
却下 ································ 51
却下理由 ···························· 53
結果 ································ 26
結語 ································ 36
欠損値 ······························ 15
研究デザイン ······················ 23
研究の限界 ························· 36
研究ロジスティックス ··········· 24
考察 ································ 35
構成要素 ······························ 9

さ行

採否結果 ···························· 50
査読者 ································ 3
サブグループ解析 ················ 30
施設内審査組織 ······················ 7
執筆順序 ······························ 9
謝辞 ································ 38
受動態 ························· 44, 96
小数点 ······························ 16
抄録 ································ 32
緒言 ································ 33
信頼区間 ···························· 29
図 ··································· 13
推敲 ··································· 4
スポンサー情報 ···················· 25

た行

前提 ··································· 2
センテンス ························· 42
測定項目の定義 ···················· 24

た行

ターゲットジャーナル ······· 8, 48
対象患者の選択 ···················· 23
対象患者背景 ······················ 27
多重性の問題 ······················ 30
多変量解析 ························· 30
中央値 ························· 16, 28
著者の資格 ························· 47
統計指標 ···························· 28
投稿先 ······························ 48

な行

2元変数 ···························· 15
日本人の論文の特徴 ·············· 42
能動態 ························· 45, 96

は行

パラグラフ ························· 42
表 ··································· 13
標準偏差 ···························· 15
表題 ································ 39
フローチャート ···················· 21
プロトコル作成 ······················ 7
文章構成 ···························· 40
平均値 ······························ 28
編集記号 ······························ 4
編集者 ································ 3
方法 ································ 22
母集団 ······························ 16

ま行

文字・図表のバランス ··········· 11

ら行

利益相反	38
臨床研究デザイン	23
倫理委員会	7
論文の構造	5

欧文

Abstract	32, 57, 77, 97, 133, 150
Acknowledgement	38, 65, 142
Authorship	47
Comment	62, 103
Conclusion	36, 85, 106, 141
Conflict of Interest	38
cover letter	48
Disclosure	142
Discussion	35, 82, 138
Figure legends	85, 106, 142
Figureの作り方	19
Impact Factor	51
Institutional Review Board (IRB)	7
Introduction	33, 58, 78, 98
Limitation	36, 105
Methods	22, 58, 80, 98, 134, 151
online投稿	48
p値	18, 29
Reference	37
Rejection	51
Results	26, 61, 81, 101, 136, 154
SD (standard deviation)	15
Sources of Funding	142
Statistical Reviewer	51
Study Flowchart	21
Tableの作り方	13
Title	39, 76, 96

175

巻末 執筆論文リスト

　今となっては，恥ずかしい論文もたくさんあるが，筆者がどの領域，どの程度の論文執筆に関わったかのかが読者にわかるように，また読者が自分の領域に関連する論文を執筆する際の参考として，以下に筆者の論文リストを挙げる．
　これらの論文での経験を通じて本書を上梓したので，当然ながら本書で書いたことと外れたものも多いが，それらも反面教師としていただきたい．

（2012年10月5現在）

[総合内科・ヘルスサービスリサーチ領域]

1) Sakuma M, Bates DW, **Morimoto T**. Clinical prediction rule to identify high risk inpatients for adverse drug events：the JADE study. ***Pharmacoepidemiol Drug Saf*** 2012 (in press).
2) Tanaka B, Sakuma M, Ohtani M, Toshiro J, Matsumura T, **Morimoto T**. Incidence and risk factors of hospital falls on long-term care wards in Japan. ***J Eval Clin Pract*** 2012；18：572-7.
3) Murata K, **Morimoto T**. A clinical database as a multi-disciplinary instructional tool. ***Gen Med*** 2012 (in press).
4) **Morimoto T**, Sakuma M, Matsui K, Kuramoto N, Toshiro J, Murakami J, Fukui T, Saito M, Hiraide A, Bates DW. Incidence of adverse drug events and medication errors in Japan：the JADE study. ***J Gen Intern Med*** 2011；26：148-53.
5) Sakuma M, **Morimoto T**. Adverse drug events due to potentially inappropriate medications. ***Arch Intern Med*** 2011；171：1959.
6) Sakuma M, **Morimoto T**, Matsui K, Seki S, Kuramoto N, Toshiro J, Murakami J, Fukui T, Saito M, Hiraide A, Bates DW. Epidemiology of potentially inappropriate medication use in elderly patients in Japanese acute care hospitals. ***Pharmacoepidemiol Drug Saf*** 2011；20：386-92.
7) Kubota Y, Yano Y, Seki S, Takada K, Sakuma M, **Morimoto T**, Akaike A, Hiraide A. Assessment of pharmacy students' communication competence using the roter interaction analysis system during objective structured clinical examinations. ***Am J Pharm Educ*** 2011；75：43.
8) Aggarwal R, Mytton OT, Derbrew M, Hananel D, Heydenburg M, Issenberg B, MacAulay C, Mancini ME, **Morimoto T**, Soper N, Ziv A, Reznick R. Training and simulation for patient safety. ***Qual Saf Health Care*** 2010；19 Suppl 2：i34-43.
9) Jha AK, Prasopa-Plaizier N, Larizgoitia I, Bates DW；Research Priority Setting Working Group of the WHO World Alliance for Patient Safety (Allegranzi B, Angood P, Bhutta Z, Davis P, Grandt D, Hamid M, Insua J, Kaitiritimba R, Khamassi S, Madiba T, **Morimoto T**, Noble D, Norton P, Pang TE, Sidorchuk R, Supachutikul A, Thomas E). Patient safety research：an overview of the global evidence. ***Qual Saf Health***

Care 2010 ; 19 : 42-7.
10) Bates DW, Larizgoitia I, Prasopa-Plaizier N, Jha AK ; Research Priority Setting Working Group of the WHO World Alliance for Patient Safety (Allegranzi B, Angood P, Bhutta Z, Davis P, Grandt D, Hamid M, Insua J, Kaitiritimba R, Khamassi S, Madiba T, **Morimoto T**, Noble D, Norton P, Pang TE, Sidorchuk R, Supachutikul A, Thomas E) . Global priorities for patient safety research. ***BMJ*** 2009 ; 338 : b1775.
11) Kuramoto N, **Morimoto T**, Kubota Y, Maeda Y, Seki S, Takada K, Hiraide A. Public perception of and willingness to perform bystander CPR in Japan. ***Resuscitation*** 2008 ; 79 : 475-81.
12) **Morimoto T**, Oguma Y, Yamazaki S, Sokejima S, Nakayama T, Fukuhara S. Gender differences in effects of physical activity on quality of life and resource utilization. ***Qual Life Res*** 2006 ; 15 : 537-46.
13) Nakamura T, Takahashi O, Matsui K, Shimizu S, Setoyama M, Nakagawa M, Fukui T, **Morimoto T**. Clinical prediction rules for bacteremia and in-hospital death based on clinical data at the time of blood withdrawal for culture : an evaluation of their development and use. ***J Eval Clin Pract*** 2006 ; 12 : 692-703.
14) Fukui T, Maeda K, Rahman M, **Morimoto T**, Saito M, Matsui K, Shimbo T. The number of lives saved and quality-adjusted life years prolonged by ticlopidine hydrochloride over the past 20 years in Japan. ***Gen Med*** 2006 ; 7 : 61-9.
15) **Morimoto T**, Gandhi TK, Fiskio JM, Seger AC, So JW, Cook EF, Fukui T, Bates DW. Development and validation of a clinical prediction rule for angiotensin-converting enzyme inhibitor-induced cough. ***J Gen Intern Med*** 2004 ; 19 : 684-91.
16) **Morimoto T**, Gandhi TK, Seger AC, Hsieh TC, Bates DW. Adverse drug events and medication errors : Detection and classification Methods. ***Qual Saf Health Care*** 2004 ; 13 : 306-14.
17) **Morimoto T**, Gandhi TK, Fiskio JM, Seger AC, So JW, Cook EF, Fukui T, Bates DW. An evaluation of risk factors for adverse drug events associated with angiotensin-converting enzyme inhibitors. ***J Eval Clin Pract*** 2004 ; 10 : 499-509.
18) **Morimoto T**, Fukui T. Utilities measured by rating scale, time trade-off, and standard gamble : review and reference for health care professionals. ***J Epidemiol*** 2002 ; 12 : 160-78.
19) Shimbo T, Nagata-Kobayashi S, **Morimoto T**, Fukui T. Quick estimation of threshold "number needed to treat". ***J Clin Epidemiol*** 2002 ; 55 : 531.
20) Koyama H, Matsui K, Goto M, Sekimoto M, Maeda K, **Morimoto T**, Hira K, Fukui T. In-patient interventions supported by Results of randomized controlled trials in Japan. ***Int J Qual Health Care*** 2002 ; 14 : 119-25.

［循環器領域］
21) Shiomi H, Nakagawa Y, **Morimoto T**, Furukawa Y, Nakano A, Shirai S, Taniguchi R, Yamaji K, Nagao K, Suyama T, Mitsuoka H, Araki M, Takashima H, Mizoguchi T, Eisawa H, Sugiyama S, Kimura T ; CREDO-Kyoto AMI investigators. Association of onset to balloon and door to balloon time with long term clinical outcome in patients with ST elevation acute myocardial infarction having primary percutaneous coronary

intervention : observational study. ***BMJ*** 2012 ; 344 : e3257.
22) Shiomi H, **Morimoto T**, Hayano M, Furukawa Y, Nakagawa Y, Tazaki J, Imai M, Yamaji K, Tada T, Natsuaki M, Saijo S, Funakoshi S, Nagao K, Hanazawa K, Ehara N, Kadota K, Iwabuchi M, Shizuta S, Abe M, Sakata R, Okabayashi H, Hanyu M, Yamazaki F, Shimamoto M, Nishiwaki N, Imoto Y, Komiya T, Horie M, Fujiwara H, Mitsudo K, Nobuyoshi M, Kita T, Kimura T ; CREDO-Kyoto PCI/CABG Registry Cohort-2 Investigators. Comparison of long-term outcome after percutaneous coronary intervention versus coronary artery bypass grafting in patients with unprotected left main coronary artery disease (from the CREDO-Kyoto PCI/CABG registry cohort-2). ***Am J Cardiol*** 2012 (in press).
23) Kimura T, **Morimoto T**, Natsuaki M, Shiomi H, Igarashi K, Kadota K, Tanabe K, Morino Y, Akasaka T, Takatsu Y, Nishikawa H, Yamamoto Y, Nakagawa Y, Hayashi Y, Iwabuchi M, Umeda H, Kawai K, Okada H, Kimura K, Simonton CA, Kozuma K. Comparison of everolimus-eluting and sirolimus-eluting coronary stents : 1-year outcomes from the randomized evaluation of sirolimus-eluting versus everolimus-eluting stent trial (RESET). ***Circulation*** 2012 (in press).
24) Kimura T, **Morimoto T**, Nakagawa Y, Kawai K, Miyazaki S, Muramatsu T, Shiode N, Namura M, Sone T, Oshima S, Nishikawa H, Hiasa Y, Hayashi Y, Nobuyoshi M, Mitudo K ; j-Cypher Registry Investigators. Very late stent thrombosis and late target lesion revascularization after sirolimus-eluting stent implantation : five-year outcome of the j-Cypher registry. ***Circulation*** 2012 ; 125 : 584-91.
25) Tokushige A, Shiomi H, **Morimoto T**, Furukawa Y, Nakagawa Y, Kadota K, Iwabuchi M, Shizuta S, Tada T, Tazaki J, Kato Y, Hayano M, Abe M, Ehara N, Inada T, Kaburagi S, Hamasaki S, Tei C, Nakashima H, Ogawa H, Tatami R, Suwa S, Takizawa A, Nohara R, Fujiwara H, Mitsudo K, Nobuyoshi M, Kita T, Kimura T ; CREDO-Kyoto PCI/CABG Registry Cohort-2 Investigators. Incidence and outcome of surgical procedures after coronary bare-metal and drug-eluting stent implantation : A report from the CREDO-Kyoto PCI/CABG registry cohort-2. ***Circ Cardiovasc Interv*** 2012 (in press).
26) Tada T, Natsuaki M, **Morimoto T**, Furukawa Y, Nakagawa Y, Byrne RA, Kastrati A, Kadota K, Iwabuchi M, Shizuta S, Tazaki J, Shiomi H, Abe M, Ehara N, Mizoguchi T, Mitsuoka H, Inada T, Araki M, Kaburagi S, Taniguchi R, Eizawa H, Nakano A, Suwa S, Takizawa A, Nohara R, Fujiwara H, Mitsudo K, Nobuyoshi M, Kita T, Kimura T ; CREDO-Kyoto PCI/CABG Registry Cohort-2 Investigators. Duration of dual antiplatelet therapy and long-term clinical outcome after coronary drug-eluting stent implantation : Landmark analyses from the CREDO-Kyoto PCI/CABG registry cohort-2. ***Circ Cardiovasc Interv*** 2012 (in press).
27) Natsuaki M, Furukawa Y, **Morimoto T**, Sakata R, Kimura T ; CREDO-Kyoto PCI/CABG Registry Cohort-2 Investigators. Renal function and effect of statin therapy on cardiovascular outcomes in patients undergoing coronary revascularization (from the CREDO-Kyoto PCI/CABG Registry Cohort-2). ***Am J Cardiol*** 2012 (in press).
28) Kato M, Kimura T, **Morimoto T**, Nishikawa H, Uchida F, Suzuki H, Hayashi Y, Kadota

K, Mitsudo K ; J-Cypher Registry Investigators. Comparison of five-year outcome of sirolimus-eluting stent implantation for chronic total occlusions versus for non-chronic total occlusion (from the j-Cypher registry). *Am J Cardiol* 2012 (in press).

29) Natsuaki M, Nakagawa Y, **Morimoto T**, Ono K, Shizuta S, Furukawa Y, Kadota K, Iwabuchi M, Kato Y, Suwa S, Inada T, Doi O, Takizawa A, Nobuyoshi M, Kita T, Kimura T ; CREDO-Kyoto PCI/CABG Registry Cohort-2 Investigators. Impact of statin therapy on late target lesion revascularization after sirolimus-eluting stent implantation (From the CREDO-Kyoto registry cohort-2). *Am J Cardiol* 2012 (in press).

30) Ozasa N, **Morimoto T**, Bao B, Furukawa Y, Nakagawa Y, Kadota K, Iwabuchi M, Shizuta S, Shiomi H, Tazaki J, Natsuaki M, Kimura T ; CREDO-Kyoto Registry Investigators. β-blockers use in patients after percutaneous coronary interventions : One size fits all? Worse outcomes in patients without myocardial infarction or heart failure. *Int J Cardiol* 2012 (in press).

31) Shizuta S, Ando K, Nobuyoshi M, Ikeda T, Yoshino H, Hiramatsu S, Kazatani Y, Yamashiro K, Okajima K, Kajiya T, Kobayashi Y, Kato T, Fujii S, Mitsudo K, Inoue K, Ito H, Haruna Y, Doi T, Nishio Y, Ozasa N, Nishiyama K, Kita T, **Morimoto T**, Kimura T ; PREVENT-SCD Investigators. Prognostic utility of T-wave alternans in a real-world population of patients with left ventricular dysfunction : the PREVENT-SCD study. *Clin Res Cardiol* 2012 (in press).

32) Ozasa N, **Morimoto T**, Bao B, Shioi T, Kimura T. Effects of machine-assisted cycling on exercise capacity and endothelial function in elderly patients with heart failure. *Circ J* 2012 (in press).

33) Soejima H, Ogawa H, **Morimoto T**, Nakayama M, Okada S, Uemura S, Kanauchi M, Doi N, Sakuma M, Jinnouchi H, Sugiyama S, Waki M, Saito Y ; JPAD Trial Investigators. Aspirin reduces cerebrovascular events in type 2 diabetic patients with poorly controlled blood pressure : Subanalysis from the JPAD trial. *Circ J* 2012 (in press).

34) Tokushige A, Shiomi H, **Morimoto T**, Ono K, Furukawa Y, Nakagawa Y, Kadota K, Iwabuchi M, Shizuta S, Tada T, Tazaki J, Kato Y, Hayano M, Abe M, Hamasaki S, Tei C, Nakashima H, Mitsudo K, Nobuyoshi M, Kita T, Kimura T. Influence of initial acute myocardial infarction presentation on the outcome of surgical procedures after coronary stent implantation : a report from the CREDO-Kyoto PCI/CABG Registry Cohort-2. *Cardiovasc Interv Ther* 2012 (in press).

35) Bao B, Ozasa N, **Morimoto T**, Furukawa Y, Nakagawa Y, Kadota K, Iwabuchi M, Shizuta S, Shiomi H, Tada T, Tazaki J, Kato Y, Hayano M, Natsuaki M, Fujiwara H, Mitsudo K, Nobuyoshi M, Kita T, Kimura T ; CREDO-Kyoto AMI Registry Investigators. Beta-blocker therapy and cardiovascular outcomes in patients who have undergone percutaneous coronary intervention after ST-elevation myocardial infarction. *Cardiovasc Interv Ther* 2012 (in press).

36) Kimura T, **Morimoto T**, Furukawa Y, Nakagawa Y, Kadota K, Iwabuchi M, Shizuta S, Shiomi H, Tada T, Tazaki J, Kato Y, Hayano M, Abe M, Tamura T, Shirotani M, Miki

S, Matsuda M, Takahashi M, Ishii K, Tanaka M, Aoyama T, Doi O, Hattori R, Tatami R, Suwa S, Takizawa A, Takatsu Y, Takahashi M, Kato H, Takeda T, Lee JD, Nohara R, Ogawa H, Tei C, Horie M, Kambara H, Fujiwara H, Mitsudo K, Nobuyoshi M, Kita T ; CREDO-Kyoto PCI/ CABG Registry Cohort-2 Investigators. Long-term safety and efficacy of sirolimus-eluting stents versus bare-metal stents in real world clinical practice in Japan. *Cardiovasc Interv Ther* 2012 (in press).

37) Kimura T, **Morimoto T**, Furukawa Y, Nakagawa Y, Kadota K, Iwabuchi M, Shizuta S, Shiomi H, Tada T, Tazaki J, Kato Y, Hayano M, Abe M, Tamura T, Shirotani M, Miki S, Matsuda M, Takahashi M, Ishii K, Tanaka M, Aoyama T, Doi O, Hattori R, Tatami R, Suwa S, Takizawa A, Takatsu Y, Takahashi M, Kato H, Takeda T, Lee JD, Nohara R, Tei C, Horie M, Kambara H, Fujiwara H, Mitsudo K, Nobuyoshi M, Kita T ; CREDO-Kyoto PCI/ CABG Registry Cohort-2 Investigators. Association of the use of proton pump inhibitors with adverse cardiovascular and bleeding outcomes after percutaneous coronary intervention in the Japanese real world clinical practice. *Cardiovasc Interv Ther* 2012 (in press).

38) Kimura T, **Morimoto T**, Nakagawa Y, Kadota K, Nozaki Y, Tada T, Take S, Shirota K, Ito A, Nakashima H, Fujita H, Kawasaki T, Inada T, Nakao K, Miyazaki S, Doi O, Isshiki T, Nobuyoshi M, Mitudo K. Antiplatelet therapy and long-term clinical outcome after sirolimus-eluting stent implantation : 5-year outcome of the j-Cypher registry. *Cardiovasc Interv Ther* 2012 (in press).

39) Nakao T, Kimura T, **Morimoto T**, Furukawa Y, Nakagawa Y, Kadota K, Nobuyoshi M, Kita T, Mitsudo K. The long-term efficacy of cilostazol in addition to dual antiplatelet therapy after sirolimus-eluting stent implantation for Japanese patients : an analysis of the 3-year follow-up outcomes from the j-Cypher registry. *Cardiovasc Interv Ther* 2012 (in press).

40) Natsuaki M, Furukawa Y, **Morimoto T**, Nakagawa Y, Ono K, Kaburagi S, Inada T, Mitsuoka H, Taniguchi R, Nakano A, Kita T, Sakata R, Kimura T ; CREDO-Kyoto PCI/CABG registry cohort-2 investigators. Intensity of statin therapy, achieved LDL-C levels and cardiovascular outcomes in Japanese patients after coronary revascularization. *Circ J* 2012 (in press).

41) Takashima H, Ozaki Y, **Morimoto T**, Kimura T, Hiro T, Miyauchi K, Nakagawa Y, Yamagishi M, Daida H, Mizuno T, Asai K, Kuroda Y, Kosaka T, Kuhara Y, Kurita A, Maeda K, Matsuzaki M ; JAPAN-ACS Investigators. Clustering of metabolic syndrome components attenuates coronary plaque regression during intensive statin therapy in patients with acute coronary syndrome - Serial intravascular ultrasound analysis from the Japan Assessment of Pitavastatin and Atorvastatin in Acute Coronary Syndrome Trial (JAPAN-ACS Trial) -. *Circ J* 2012 (in press).

42) Miyauchi K, Daida H, **Morimoto T**, Hiro T, Kimura T, Nakagawa Y, Yamagishi M, Ozaki Y, Kadota K, Kimura K, Hirayama A, Kimura K, Hasegawa Y, Uchiyama S, Matsuzaki M ; JAPAN-ACS Investigators. Reverse vessel remodeling but not coronary plaque regression could predict future cardiovascular events in ACS patients with intensive statin therapy. *Circ J* 2012 (in press).

43) Takami T, Yamano S, Okada S, Sakuma M, **Morimoto T**, Hashimoto H, Somekawa S, Saito Y. Major risk factors for the appearance of white-matter lesions on MRI in hypertensive patients with controlled blood pressure. *Vasc Health Risk Manag* 2012 ; 8 : 169-76.
44) Natsuaki M, **Morimoto T**, Furukawa Y, Nakagawa Y, Kadota K, Iwabuchi M, Shizuta S, Shiomi H, Kimura T. Comparison of 3-year clinical outcomes after transradial versus transfemoral percutaneous coronary intervention. *Cardiovasc Interv Ther* 2012 ; 27 : 84-92.
45) Hibi K, Kimura T, Kimura K, **Morimoto T**, Hiro T, Miyauchi K, Nakagawa Y, Yamagishi M, Ozaki Y, Saito S, Yamaguchi T, Daida H, Matsuzaki M ; JAPAN-ACS Investigators. Clinically evident polyvascular disease and regression of coronary atherosclerosis after intensive statin therapy in patients with acute coronary syndrome : Serial intravascular ultrasound from the Japanese assessment of pitavastatin and atorvastatin in acute coronary syndrome (JAPAN-ACS) trial. *Atherosclerosis* 2011 ; 219 : 743-749.
46) Okada S, **Morimoto T**, Ogawa H, Kanauchi M, Nakayama M, Uemura S, Doi N, Jinnouchi H, Waki M, Soejima H, Sakuma M, Saito Y ; Japanese Primary Prevention of Atherosclerosis with Aspirin for Diabetes Trial Investigators. Differential effect of low-dose aspirin for primary prevention of atherosclerotic events in diabetes management : a subanalysis of the JPAD trial. *Diabetes Care* 2011 ; 34 : 1277-83.
47) Saito Y, **Morimoto T**, Ogawa H, Nakayama M, Uemura S, Doi N, Jinnouchi H, Waki M, Soejima H, Sugiyama S, Okada S, Akai Y ; Japanese Primary Prevention of Atherosclerosis with Aspirin for Diabetes Trial Investigators. Low-dose aspirin therapy in patients with type 2 diabetes and reduced glomerular filtration rate : subanalysis from the JPAD trial. *Diabetes Care* 2011 ; 34 : 280-5.
48) Doi T, Makiyama T, **Morimoto T**, Haruna Y, Tsuji K, Ohno S, Akao M, Takahashi Y, Kimura T, Horie M. A novel KCNJ2 nonsense mutation, S369X, impedes trafficking and causes a limited form of Andersen-Tawil syndrome. *Circ Cardiovasc Genet* 2011 ; 4 : 253-60.
49) Kishi K, Kimura T, **Morimoto T**, Namura M, Muramatsu T, Nishikawa H, Hiasa Y, Isshiki T, Nobuyoshi M, Mitsudo K ; j-Cypher Registry Investigators. Sirolimus-eluting stent implantation for ostial left anterior descending coronary artery lesions : three-year outcome from the j-Cypher Registry. *Circ Cardiovasc Interv* 2011 ; 4 : 362-70.
50) Morino Y, Abe M, **Morimoto T**, Kimura T, Hayashi Y, Muramatsu T, Ochiai M, Noguchi Y, Kato K, Shibata Y, Hiasa Y, Doi O, Yamashita T, Hinohara T, Tanaka H, Mitsudo K ; J-CTO Registry Investigators. Predicting successful guidewire crossing through chronic total occlusion of native coronary lesions within 30 minutes : the J-CTO (Multicenter CTO Registry in Japan) score as a difficulty grading and time assessment tool. *JACC Cardiovasc Interv* 2011 ; 4 : 213-21.
51) Tada T, Kimura T, **Morimoto T**, Ono K, Furukawa Y, Nakagawa Y, Nakashima H, Ito A, Siode N, Namura M, Inoue N, Nishikawa H, Nakao K, Mitsudo K ; j-Cypher Registry Investigators. Comparison of three-year clinical outcomes after sirolimus-eluting stent

implantation among insulin-treated diabetic, non-insulin-treated diabetic, and non-diabetic patients from j-Cypher registry. *Am J Cardiol* 2011 ; 107 : 1155-62.

52) Tamura T, Kimura T, **Morimoto T**, Nakagawa Y, Furukawa Y, Kadota K, Tatami R, Kawai K, Sone T, Miyazaki S, Mitsudo K ; j-Cypher Registry Investigators. Three-year outcome of sirolimus-eluting stent implantation in coronary bifurcation lesions : the provisional side branch stenting approach versus the elective two-stent approach. *EuroIntervention* 2011 ; 7 : 588-96.

53) Toyofuku M, Kimura T, **Morimoto T**, Hayashi Y, Shiode N, Okimoto T, Otsuka M, Tamekiyo H, Tamura T, Kadota K, Inoue K, Mitsudo K ; j-Cypher Registry investigators. Comparison of target-lesion revascularisation between left main coronary artery bifurcations and left anterior descending coronary artery bifurcations using the one and two stent approach with sirolimus-eluting stents. *EuroIntervention* 2011 ; 7 : 796-804.

54) Imai M, Kadota K, Goto T, Fujii S, Yamamoto H, Fuku Y, Hosogi S, Hirono A, Tanaka H, Tada T, **Morimoto T**, Shiomi H, Kozuma K, Inoue K, Suzuki N, Kimura T, Mitsudo K. Incidence, risk factors, and clinical sequelae of angiographic peri-stent contrast staining after sirolimus-eluting stent implantation. *Circulation* 2011 ; 123 : 2382-91.

55) Funakoshi S, Furukawa Y, Ehara N, **Morimoto T**, Kaji S, Yamamuro A, Kinoshita M, Kitai T, Kim K, Tani T, Kobori A, Nasu M, Okada Y, Kita T, Kimura T ; CREDO-Kyoto Investigators. Clinical characteristics and outcomes of Japanese women undergoing coronary revascularization therapy. *Circ J* 2011 ; 75 : 1358-67.

56) Natsuaki M, Furukawa Y, **Morimoto T**, Nakagawa Y, Akao M, Ono K, Shioi T, Shizuta S, Sakata R, Okabayashi H, Nishiwaki N, Komiya T, Suwa S, Kimura T. Impact of diabetes on cardiovascular outcomes in hemodialysis patients undergoing coronary revascularization. *Circ J* 2011 ; 75 : 1616-25.

57) Shiomi H, Tamura T, Niki S, Tada T, Tazaki J, Toma M, Ono K, Shioi T, **Morimoto T**, Akao M, Furukawa Y, Nakagawa Y, Kimura T. Inter- and intra-observer variability for assessment of the synergy between percutaneous coronary intervention with TAXUS and cardiac surgery (SYNTAX) score and association of the SYNTAX score with clinical outcome in patients undergoing unprotected left main stenting in the real world. *Circ J* 2011 ; 75 : 1130-7.

58) Soejima H, **Morimoto T**, Saito Y, Ogawa H. Aspirin for the primary prevention of cardiovascular events in patients with peripheral artery disease or diabetes mellitus. Analyses from the JPAD, POPADAD and AAA trials. *Thromb Haemost* 2010 ; 104 : 1085-8.

59) Ozasa N, **Morimoto T**, Furukawa Y, Hamazaki H, Kita T, Kimura T. Six-minute walk distance in Japanese healthy adults. *Gen Med* 2010 ; 11 : 25-30.

60) Kimura T, **Morimoto T**, Kozuma K, Honda Y, Kume T, Aizawa T, Mitsudo K, Miyazaki S, Yamaguchi T, Hiyoshi E, Nishimura E, Isshiki T ; RESTART Investigators. Comparisons of baseline demographics, clinical presentation, and long-term outcome among patients with early, late, and very late stent thrombosis of sirolimus-eluting stents : Observations from the Registry of Stent Thrombosis for

Review and Reevaluation (RESTART). *Circulation* 2010 ; 122 : 52-61.
61) Abe M, Kimura T, **Morimoto T**, Taniguchi T, Yamanaka F, Nakao K, Yagi N, Kokubu N, Kasahara Y, Kataoka Y, Otsuka Y, Kawamura A, Miyazaki S, Nakao K, Horiuchi K, Ito A, Hoshizaki H, Kawaguchi R, Setoguchi M, Inada T, Kishi K, Sakamoto H, Morioka N, Imai M, Shiomi H, Nonogi H, Mitsudo K ; j-Cypher Registry Investigators. Sirolimus-eluting stent versus balloon angioplasty for sirolimus-eluting stent restenosis : Insights from the j-Cypher Registry. *Circulation* 2010 ; 122 : 42-51.
62) Yamaji K, Kimura T, **Morimoto T**, Nakagawa Y, Inoue K, Soga Y, Arita T, Shirai S, Ando K, Kondo K, Sakai K, Goya M, Iwabuchi M, Yokoi H, Nosaka H, Nobuyoshi M. Very long-term (15 to 20 years) clinical and angiographic outcome after coronary bare metal stent implantation. *Circ Cardiovasc Interv* 2010 ; 3 : 468-75.
63) Ozasa N, Kimura T, **Morimoto T**, Hou H, Tamura T, Shizuta S, Nakagawa Y, Furukawa Y, Hayashi Y, Nakao K, Matsuzaki M, Nobuyoshi M, Mitsudo K ; j-Cypher Registry Investigators. Lack of effect of oral beta-blocker therapy at discharge on long-term clinical outcomes of ST-segment elevation acute myocardial infarction after primary percutaneous coronary intervention. *Am J Cardiol* 2010 ; 106 : 1225-33.
64) Kawaguchi R, Kimura T, **Morimoto T**, Oshima S, Hoshizaki H, Kawai K, Shiode N, Hiasa Y, Mitsudo K ; j-Cypher Registry Investigators. Safety and efficacy of sirolimus-eluting stent implantation in patients with acute coronary syndrome in the real world. *Am J Cardiol* 2010 ; 106 : 1550-60.
65) Nakagawa Y, Kimura T, **Morimoto T**, Nomura M, Saku K, Haruta S, Muramatsu T, Nobuyoshi M, Kadota K, Fujita H, Tatami R, Shiode N, Nishikawa H, Shibata Y, Miyazaki S, Murata Y, Honda T, Kawasaki T, Doi O, Hiasa Y, Hayashi Y, Matsuzaki M, Mitsudo K ; j-Cypher Registry Investigators. Incidence and risk factors of late target lesion revascularization after sirolimus-eluting stent implantation (3-year follow-up of the j-Cypher Registry). *Am J Cardiol* 2010 ; 106 : 329-36.
66) Ohashi T, Shibata R, **Morimoto T**, Kanashiro M, Ishii H, Ichimiya S, Hiro T, Miyauchi K, Nakagawa Y, Yamagishi M, Ozaki Y, Kimura T, Daida H, Murohara T, Matsuzaki M. Correlation between circulating adiponectin levels and coronary plaque regression during aggressive lipid-lowering therapy in patients with acute coronary syndrome : Subgroup analysis of JAPAN-ACS study. *Atherosclerosis* 2010 ; 212 : 237-42.
67) Arai H, Hiro T, Kimura T, **Morimoto T**, Miyauchi K, Nakagawa Y, Yamagishi M, Ozaki Y, Kimura K, Saito S, Yamaguchi T, Daida H, Matsuzaki M ; JAPAN-ACS Investigators. More intensive lipid lowering is associated with regression of coronary atherosclerosis in diabetic patients with acute coronary syndrome--sub-analysis of JAPAN-ACS study. *J Atheroscler Thromb* 2010 ; 17 : 1096-107.
68) Nishiyama K, **Morimoto T**, Furukawa Y, Nakagawa Y, Ehara N, Taniguchi R, Ozasa N, Saito N, Hoshino K, Touma M, Tamura T, Haruna Y, Shizuta S, Doi T, Fukushima M, Kita T, Kimura T. Chronic obstructive pulmonary disease-An independent risk factor for long-term cardiac and cardiovascular mortality in patients with ischemic heart disease. *Int J Cardiol* 2010 ; 143 : 178-83.
69) Nishiyama K, Shizuta S, Doi T, **Morimoto T**, Kimura T. Sudden cardiac death after

PCI and CABG in the bare-metal stent era : Incidence, prevalence, and predictors. ***Int J Cardiol*** 2010 ; 144 : 263-6.
70) Ehara N, **Morimoto T**, Furukawa Y, Shizuta S, Taniguchi R, Nakagawa Y, Hoshino K, Saito N, Doi T, Haruna Y, Ozasa N, Imai Y, Teramukai S, Fukushima M, Kita T, Kimura T. Effect of baseline glycemic level on long-term cardiovascular outcomes after coronary revascularization therapy in patients with type 2 diabetes mellitus treated with hypoglycemic agents. ***Am J Cardiol*** 2010 ; 105 : 960-6.
71) Shirai S, Kimura T, Nobuyoshi M, **Morimoto T**, Ando K, Soga Y, Yamaji K, Kondo K, Sakai K, Arita T, Goya M, Iwabuchi M, Yokoi H, Nosaka H, Mitsudo K ; j-Cypher Registry Investigators. Impact of multiple and long sirolimus-eluting stent implantation on 3-year clinical outcomes in the j-Cypher Registry. ***JACC Cardiovasc Interv*** 2010 ; 3 : 180-8.
72) Morino Y, Kimura T, Hayashi Y, Muramatsu T, Ochiai M, Noguchi Y, Kato K, Shibata Y, Hiasa Y, Doi O, Yamashita T, **Morimoto T**, Abe M, Hinohara T, Mitsudo K ; J-CTO Registry Investigators. In-hospital outcomes of contemporary percutaneous coronary intervention in patients with chronic total occlusion insights from the J-CTO Registry (Multicenter CTO Registry in Japan). ***JACC Cardiovasc Interv*** 2010 ; 3 : 143-51.
73) Hiro T, Kimura T, **Morimoto T**, Miyauchi K, Nakagawa Y, Yamagishi M, Ozaki Y, Kimura K, Saito S, Yamaguchi T, Daida H, Matsuzaki M ; JAPAN-ACS Investigators. Diabetes mellitus is a major negative determinant of coronary plaque regression during statin therapy in patients with acute coronary syndrome--serial intravascular ultrasound observations from the Japan Assessment of Pitavastatin and Atorvastatin in Acute Coronary Syndrome Trial (the JAPAN-ACS Trial). ***Circ J*** 2010 ; 74 : 1165-74.
74) Hiro T, Kimura T, **Morimoto T**, Miyauchi K, Nakagawa Y, Yamagishi M, Ozaki Y, Kimura K, Saito S, Yamaguchi T, Daida H, Matsuzaki M. Reply : Noninferiority of pitavastatin in intravascular ultrasound findings. ***J Am Coll Cardiol*** 2010 ; 55 : 263.
75) Hamasu S, **Morimoto T**, Kuramoto N, Horiguchi M, Iwami T, Nishiyama C, Takada K, Kubota Y, Seki S, Maeda Y, Sakai Y, Hiraide A. Effects of BLS training on factors associated with attitude toward CPR in college students. ***Resuscitation*** 2009 ; 80 : 359-64.
76) Kimura T, **Morimoto T**, Nakagawa Y, Tamura T, Kadota K, Yasumoto H, Nishikawa H, Hiasa Y, Muramatsu T, Meguro T, Inoue N, Honda H, Hayashi Y, Miyazaki S, Oshima S, Honda T, Shiode N, Namura M, Sone T, Nobuyoshi M, Kita T, Mitsudo K ; j-Cypher Registry Investigators. Antiplatelet therapy and stent thrombosis after sirolimus-eluting stent implantation. ***Circulation*** 2009 ; 119 : 987-95.
77) Hiro T, Kimura T, **Morimoto T**, Miyauchi K, Nakagawa Y, Yamagishi M, Ozaki Y, Kimura K, Saito S, Yamaguchi T, Daida H, Matsuzaki M ; JAPAN-ACS Investigators. Effect of intensive statin therapy on regression of coronary atherosclerosis in patients with acute coronary syndrome : a multicenter randomized trial evaluated by volumetric intravascular ultrasound using pitavastatin versus atorvastatin (JAPAN-ACS [Japan assessment of pitavastatin and atorvastatin in acute coronary syndrome]

study). ***J Am Coll Cardiol*** 2009 ; 54 : 293-302.
78) Toyofuku M, Kimura T, **Morimoto T**, Hayashi Y, Ueda H, Kawai K, Nozaki Y, Hiramatsu S, Miura A, Yokoi Y, Toyoshima S, Nakashima H, Haze K, Tanaka M, Take S, Saito S, Isshiki T, Mitsudo K ; j-Cypher Registry Investigators. Three-year outcomes after sirolimus-eluting stent implantation for unprotected left main coronary artery disease : Insights from the j-Cypher registry. ***Circulation*** 2009 ; 120 : 1866-74.
79) Abe M, Kimura T, **Morimoto T**, Furukawa Y, Kita T. Incidence of and risk factors for contrast-induced nephropathy after cardiac catheterization in Japanese patients. ***Circ J*** 2009 ; 73 : 1518-22.
80) Furukawa Y, Ehara N, Taniguchi R, Haruna Y, Ozasa N, Saito N, Doi T, Hoshino K, Tamura T, Shizuta S, Abe M, Toma M, **Morimoto T**, Teramukai S, Fukushima M, Kita T, Kimura T ; CREDO-Kyoto Investigators. Coronary risk factor profile and prognostic factors for young Japanese patients undergoing coronary revascularization. ***Circ J*** 2009 ; 73 : 1459-65.
81) Hoshino K, Horiuchi H, Tada T, Tazaki J, Nishi E, Kawato M, Ikeda T, Yamamoto H, Akao M, Furukawa Y, Shizuta S, Toma M, Tamura T, Saito N, Doi T, Ozasa N, Jinnai T, Takahashi K, Watanabe H, Yoshikawa Y, Nishimoto N, Ouchi C, **Morimoto T**, Kita T, Kimura T. Clopidogrel resistance in Japanese patients scheduled for percutaneous coronary intervention. ***Circ J*** 2009 ; 73 : 336-42.
82) Kimura T, **Morimoto T**, Furukawa Y, Nakagawa Y, Shizuta S, Ehara N, Taniguchi R, Doi T, Nishiyama K, Ozasa N, Saito N, Hoshino K, Mitsuoka H, Abe M, Toma M, Tamura T, Haruna Y, Imai Y, Teramukai S, Fukushima M, Kita T. Long-term outcomes of coronary-artery bypass graft surgery versus percutaneous coronary intervention for multivessel coronary artery disease in the bare-metal stent era. ***Circulation*** 2008 ; 118 : S199-209.
83) Ozasa N, **Morimoto T**, Furukawa Y, Shizuta S, Nishiyama K, Kita T, Kimura T. Effects of ICD implantation on quality-adjusted life years in patients with congestive heart failure. ***Int J Cardiol*** 2008 ; 123 : 213-6.
84) Ogawa H, Nakayama M, **Morimoto T**, Uemura S, Kanauchi M, Doi N, Jinnouchi H, Sugiyama S, Saito Y ; Japanese Primary Prevention of Atherosclerosis with Aspirin for Diabetes (JPAD) Trial Investigators. Low-dose aspirin for primary prevention of atherosclerotic events in patients with type 2 diabetes : a randomized controlled trial. ***JAMA*** 2008 ; 300 : 2134-41.
85) Furukawa Y, Taniguchi R, Ehara N, Ozasa N, Haruna Y, Saito N, Doi T, Hoshino K, Shizuta S, **Morimoto T**, Imai Y, Teramukai S, Fukushima M, Kita T, Kimura T ; CREDO-Kyoto Investigators. Better survival with statin administration after revascularization therapy in Japanese patients with coronary artery disease. ***Circ J*** 2008 ; 72 : 1937-45.
86) Yamamoto H, Takahashi K, Watanabe H, Yoshikawa Y, Shirakawa R, Higashi T, Kawato M, Ikeda T, Tabuchi A, **Morimoto T**, Kita T, Horiuchi H. Evaluation of the antiplatelet effects of cilostazol, a phosphodiesterase 3 inhibitor, by VASP phosphorylation and platelet aggregation. ***Circ J*** 2008 ; 72 : 1844-51.

87) Ozasa N, Furukawa Y, **Morimoto T**, Tadamura E, Kita T, Kimura T. Relation among left ventricular mass, insulin resistance, and hemodynamic parameters in type 2 diabetes. *Hypertens Res* 2008 ; 31 : 425-32.
88) Tabuchi A, Taniguchi R, Takahashi K, Kondo H, Kawato M, **Morimoto T**, Kimura T, Kita T, Horiuchi H. Action of aspirin on whole blood-aggregation evaluated by the screen filtration pressure Methods. *Circ J.* 2008 ; 72 : 420-6.
89) **Morimoto T**, Matsui K. Aspirin for primary prevention in Japan. *Intern Med* 2007 ; 46 : 1281.
90) **Morimoto T**, Nakayama M, Saito Y, Ogawa H. Aspirin for primary prevention of atherosclerotic disease in Japan. *J Atheroscler Thromb* 2007 ; 14 : 159-66.
91) Nishio Y, Sato Y, Taniguchi R, Shizuta S, Doi T, **Morimoto T**, Kimura T, Kita T. Cardiac troponin T vs other biochemical markers in patients with congestive heart failure. *Circ J* 2007 ; 71 : 631-5.
92) Miyauchi K, Kimura T, **Morimoto T**, Nakagawa Y, Yamagishi M, Ozaki Y, Hiro T, Daida H, Matsuzaki M. Japan assessment of pitavastatin and atorvastatin in acute coronary syndrome (JAPAN-ACS) : rationale and design. *Circ J* 2006 ; 70 : 1624-8.
93) **Morimoto T**, Fukui T, Lee TH, Matsui K. Application of U.S. guidelines in other countries : Aspirin for the primary prevention of cardiovascular events in Japan. *Am J Med* 2004 ; 117 : 459-68.
94) **Morimoto T**, Hayashino Y, Shimbo T, Izumi T, Fukui T. Is B-type natriuretic peptide-guided heart failure management cost-effective? *Int J Cardiol* 2004 ; 96 : 177-81.
95) Hayashino Y, Nagata-Kobayashi S, **Morimoto T**, Maeda K, Shimbo T, Fukui T. Cost-effectiveness of screening for coronary artery disease in asymptomatic patients with type 2 diabetes and additional atherogenic risk factors. *J Gen Intern Med* 2004 ; 19 : 1181-91.

[小児領域]
96) Kusunoki T, **Morimoto T**, Sakuma M, Mukaida K, Yasumi T, Nishikomori R, Heike T. Effect of eczema on the association between season of birth and food allergy in Japanese children. *Pediatr Int* 2012 (in press).
97) Kusunoki T, Mukaida K, **Morimoto T**, Sakuma M, Yasumi T, Nishikomori R, Heike T. Birth oder effect onf childhood food allerty. *Pediatr Allergy Immunol* 2012 (in press).
98) Kusunoki T, **Morimoto T**, Sakuma M, Mukaida K, Yasumi T, Nishikomori R, Fujii T, Heike T. Total and low-density lipoprotein cholesterol levels are associated with atopy in schoolchildren. *J Pediatr* 2011 ; 158 : 334-6.
99) Kusunoki T, **Morimoto T**, Nishikomori R, Yasumi T, Heike T, Mukaida K, Fujii T, Nakahata T. Breastfeeding and the prevalence of allergic diseases in schoolchildren : Does reverse causation matter? *Pediatr Allergy Immunol* 2010 ; 21 : 60-6.
100) Mukaida K, Kusunoki T, **Morimoto T**, Yasumi T, Nishikomori R, Heike T, Fujii T, Nakahata T. The effect of past food avoidance due to allergic symptoms on the growth of children at school age. *Allergol Int* 2010 ; 59 : 369-74.
101) Kusunoki T, **Morimoto T**, Nishikomori R, Heike T, Fujii T, Nakahata T. Allergic

status of schoolchildren with food allergy to eggs, milk or wheat in infancy. ***Pediatr Allergy Immunol*** 2009 ; 20 : 642-7.

102) Kusunoki T, **Morimoto T**, Nishikomori R, Yasumi T, Heike T, Fujii T, Nakahata T. Changing prevalence and severity of childhood allergic diseases in kyoto, Japan, from 1996 to 2006. ***Allergol Int*** 2009 ; 58 : 543-8.

103) Kusunoki T, **Morimoto T**, Nishikomori R, Heike T, Ito M, Hosoi S, Nakahata T. Obesity and the prevalence of allergic diseases in schoolchildren. ***Pediatr Allergy Immunol*** 2008 ; 19 : 527-34.

104) Okamoto S, Kamiya I, Kishida K, Shimakawa T, Fukui T, **Morimoto T**. Experience with oseltamivir for infants younger than 1 year old in Japan. ***Pediatr Infect Dis J*** 2005 ; 24 : 575-576.

[呼吸器領域]

105) Ikai H, **Morimoto T**, Shimbo T, Imanaka Y, Koike K. Impact of postgraduate education on physician practice for community-acquired pneumonia. ***J Eval Clin Pract*** 2012 (in press).

106) Oga T, Chin K, Tabuchi A, Kawato M, **Morimoto T**, Takahashi K, Handa T, Takahashi K, Taniguchi R, Kondo H, Mishima M, Kita T, Horiuchi H. Effects of obstructive sleep apnea with intermittent hypoxia on platelet aggregability. ***J Atheroscler Thromb*** 2009 ; 16 : 862-9.

107) **Morimoto T**, Shimbo T, Noguchi Y, Koyama H, Sasaki Y, Nishiwaki K, Fukui T. Effects of timing of thoracoscopic surgery for primary spontaneous pneumothorax on prognosis and costs. ***Am J Surg*** 2004 ; 187 : 767-74.

108) **Morimoto T**, Fukui T, Koyama H, Noguchi Y, Shimbo T. Optimal strategy for the first episode of primary spontaneous pneumothorax in young men. A decision analysis. ***J Gen Intern Med*** 2002 ; 17 : 193-202.

[消化器領域]

109) **Morimoto T**, Noguchi Y, Sakai T, Shimbo T, Fukui T. Acute pancreatitis and the role of histamine-2 receptor antagonists : a meta-analysis of randomized controlled trials of cimetidine. ***Eur J Gastroenterol Hepatol*** 2002 ; 14 : 679-86.

[腎臓・泌尿器領域]

110) Taji Y, Kuwahara T, Shikata S, **Morimoto T**. Meta-analysis of antiplatelet therapy for IgA nephropathy. ***Clin Exp Nephrol*** 2006 ; 10 : 268-73.

111) Taji Y, **Morimoto T**, Fukuhara S, Fukui T, Kuwahara T. Effects of low dialysate calcium concentration on health-related quality of life in hemodialysis patients. ***Clin Exp Nephrol*** 2005 ; 9 : 153-7.

112) Taji Y, **Morimoto T**, Okada K, Fukuhara S, Fukui T, Kuwahara T. Effects of intravenous ascorbic acid on erythropoiesis and quality of life in unselected hemodialysis patients. ***J Nephrol*** 2004 ; 17 : 537-43.

[内分泌・代謝領域]

113) Majima T, Komatsu Y, Doi K, Takagi C, Shigemoto M, Fukao A, **Morimoto T**, Corners J, Nakao K. Negative correlation between bone mineral density and TSH receptor antibodies in male patients with untreated Graves' disease. ***Osteoporos Int*** 2006 ;

17 : 1103-10.
114) Majima T, Komatsu Y, Doi K, Takagi C, Shigemoto M, Fukao A, **Morimoto T**, Corners J, Nakao K. Clinical significance of risedronate for osteoporosis in the initial treatment of male patients with Graves' disease. *J Bone Miner Metab* 2006 ; 24 : 105-13.

[脳・神経領域]

115) Shimbo T, Goto M, **Morimoto T**, Hira K, Takemura M, Matsui K, Yoshida A, Fukui T. Association between patient education and health-related quality of life in patients with Parkinson's disease. *Qual Life Res* 2004 ; 13 : 81-89.

116) **Morimoto T**, Shimbo T, Orav JE, Matsui K, Goto M, Takemura M, Hira K, Fukui T. Impact of social functioning and vitality on preference for life in patients with Parkinson's disease. *Mov Disord* 2003 ; 18 : 171-5.

[外科領域]

117) Ohe H, Waki K, Yoshitomi M, **Morimoto T**, Nafady-Hego H, Satoda N, Li Y, Zhao X, Sakaguchi S, Uemoto S, Bishop GA, Koshiba T. Factors affecting operational tolerance after pediatric living-donor liver transplantation : Impact of early post-transplant events and HLA match. *Transpl Int* 2012 ; 25 : 97-106.

[整形外科領域]

118) Goto K, Akiyama H, Kawanabe K, So K, **Morimoto T**, Nakamura T. Long-term Results of cemented total hip arthroplasty for dysplasia, with structural autograft fixed with poly-L-lactic acid screws. *J Arthroplasty* 2009 ; 24 : 1146-51.

119) Goto K, Kawanabe K, Akiyama H, **Morimoto T**, Nakamura T. Clinical and radiological evaluation of revision hip arthroplasty using the cement-in-cement technique. *J Bone Joint Surg* 2008 ; 90 : 1013-8.

[感覚器領域]

120) Nomura K, Nakao M, **Morimoto T**. Effects of smoking on hearing loss : Quality assessment and meta-analysis. *Prev Med* 2005 ; 40 : 138-44.

[アレルギー・免疫領域]

121) Tanaka N, Izawa K, Saito MK, Sakuma M, Oshima K, Ohara O, Nishikomori R, **Morimoto T**, Kambe N, Goldbach-Mansky R, Aksentijevich I, de Saint Basile G, Neven B, van Gijn M, Frenkel J, Aróstegui JI, Yagüe J, Merino R, Ibañez M, Pontillo A, Takada H, Imagawa T, Kawai T, Yasumi T, Nakahata T, Heike T. High incidence of NLRP3 somatic mosaicism in patients with chronic infantile neurologic, cutaneous, articular syndrome : Results of an international multicenter collaborative study. *Arthritis Rheum* 2011 ; 63 : 3625-32.

[がん領域]

122) Nomura K, Kawasugi K, **Morimoto T**. Cost-effectiveness analysis of antifungal treatment for patients on chemotherapy. *Eur J Cancer Care* 2006 ; 15 : 44-50.

[基礎医学領域]

123) Lee J, Kanatsu-Shinohara M, Ogonuki N, Miki H, Inoue K, **Morimoto T**, Morimoto H, Ogura A, Shinohara T. Heritable imprinting defect caused by epigenetic abnormalities in mouse spermatogonial stem cells. *Biol Reprod* 2009 ; 80 : 518-27.

124) Kanatsu-Shinohara M, Inoue K, Miki H, Ogonuki N, Takehashi M, **Morimoto T**, Ogura

A, Shinohara T. Clonal origin of germ cell colonies after spermatogonial transplantation in mice. ***Biol Reprod*** 2006 ; 75 : 68-74.
125) Kanatsu-Shinohara M, **Morimoto T**, Toyokuni S, Shinohara T. Regulation of mouse spermatogonial stem cell self-renewing division by the pituitary gland. ***Biol Reprod*** 2004 ; 70 : 1731-7.
126) Kanatsu-Shinohara M, Toyokuni S, **Morimoto T**, Matsui S, Honjo T, Shinohara T. Functional assessment of self-renewal activity of male germline stem cells following cytotoxic damage and serial transplantation. ***Biol Reprod*** 2003 ; 68 : 1801-7.
127) Yagi T, **Morimoto T**, Takebe H. Correlation of (6-4) photoproduct formation with transforming mutations in UV-irradiated Ha-ras. ***Carcinogenesis*** 1995 ; 16 : 689-95.

森本　剛 略歴

平成 7 (1995) 年		京都大学医学部 卒業
		京都大学医学部附属病院総合診療部，市立舞鶴市民病院内科，国立京都病院総合内科，Brigham and Women's 病院総合診療科を経て
平成 14 (2002) 年		Harvard 大学公衆衛生大学院公衆衛生修士課程 修了
平成 16 (2004) 年		京都大学大学院医学研究科内科系専攻博士課程 修了
	同年	京都大学医学部附属病院総合診療科 助手
平成 17 (2005) 年		京都大学大学院医学研究科医学教育推進センター 講師
平成 20 (2008) 年		慶應義塾大学大学院経営管理研究科科目履修生 修了
平成 23 (2011) 年		近畿大学医学部救急総合診療センター 教授
平成 25 (2013) 年		兵庫医科大学内科学総合診療科 教授

中山書店の出版物に関する情報は，小社サポートページを御覧ください．
http://www.nakayamashoten.co.jp/bookss/define/support/support.html

査読者が教える
採用される医学論文の書き方

2013年5月1日　初版第1刷発行©　〔検印省略〕
2013年8月5日　　　第2刷発行
2014年5月30日　　　第3刷発行

著　者　——　森本　剛

発行者　——　平田　直

発行所　——　株式会社 中山書店
　　　　　　〒113-8666　東京都文京区白山 1-25-14
　　　　　　TEL 03-3813-1100（代表）　振替 00130-5-196565
　　　　　　http://www.nakayamashoten.co.jp/

DTP　——　クニメディア株式会社

装丁　——　臼井弘志（公和図書デザイン室）

印刷・製本　——　三報社印刷株式会社

ISBN978-4-521-73701-0
Published by Nakayama Shoten Co., Ltd.　　　　　　　　　　Printed in Japan
落丁・乱丁の場合はお取り替え致します

・本書の複製権・上映権・譲渡権・公衆送信権（送信可能化権を含む）は株式会社中山書店が保有します．

・JCOPY ＜（社）出版者著作権管理機構 委託出版物＞
本書の無断複写は著作権法上での例外を除き禁じられています．複写される場合は，そのつど事前に，(社)出版者著作権管理機構（電話 03-3513-6969, FAX 03-3513-6979, e-mail: info@jcopy.or.jp）の許諾を得てください．

・本書をスキャン・デジタルデータ化するなどの複製を無許諾で行う行為は，著作権法上での限られた例外（「私的使用のための複製」など）を除き著作権法違反となります．なお，大学・病院・企業などにおいて，内部的に業務上使用する目的で上記の行為を行うことは，私的使用には該当せず違法です．また私的使用のためであっても，代行業者等の第三者に依頼して使用する本人以外の者が上記の行為を行うことは違法です．

あなたの知識はマイナスだらけ!?
統計がとても身近になる!

p値依存症のアナタに捧ぐ

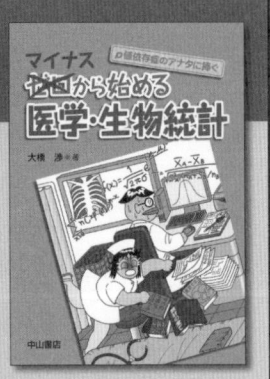

マイナスから始める医学・生物統計

A5判／並製／160頁
定価（本体3,200円＋税）
ISBN978-4-521-73479-8

"統計"と聞いただけで身構えてしまう人たちのために医学・生物統計の意味とおもしろさを，日常的な例とたとえで分かりやすく解説．読み終わったときにはあなたの統計学が記念すべき一歩をしるす！

著●大橋 渉

独自の視点で医学生物統計の基本的考え方を解説

CONTENTS

第1章 統計学あれこれ
1. 確率・統計の存在感
2. 統計学は難しい？

第2章 データをどう扱う？
1. データ四方山話
2. データの種類と処理方法

第3章 統計的推定・検定とは？
1. p値と検定
2. 依存症と戦う？

第4章 分布と検定
1. それでも理論は無視できない！
2. 分布と検定

第5章 医学研究のデザインとは？
1. 医学・生物統計学とは
2. バイアスだらけ？
3. 研究デザインの重要性

ユーモアあふれる文体で，楽しく読める

中山書店　〒113-8666 東京都文京区白山1-25-14　TEL 03-3813-1100　FAX 03-3816-1015
http://www.nakayamashoten.co.jp/